Life Without Diabetes

The Cookbook

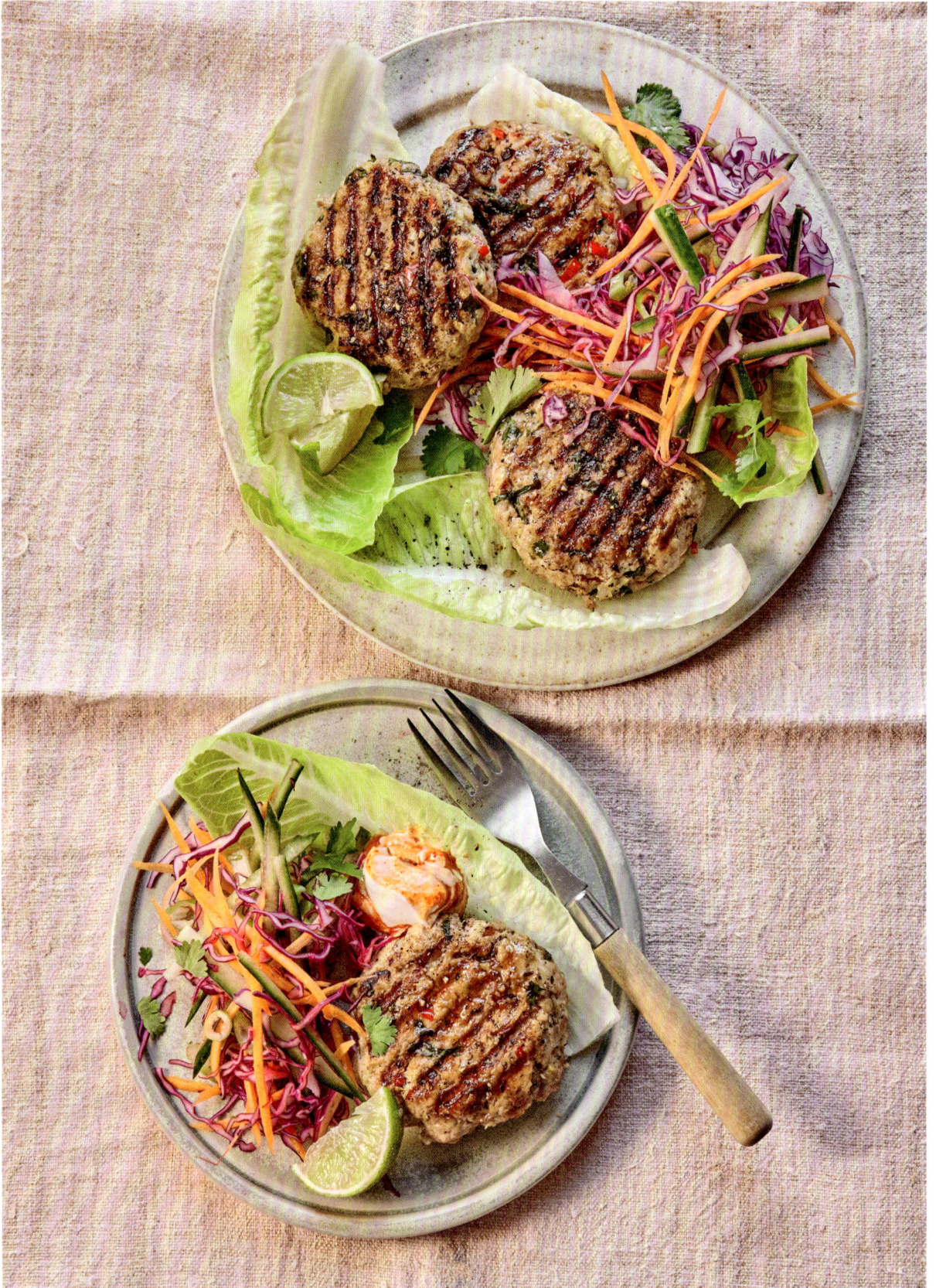

85 SIMPLE & DELICIOUS RECIPES FOR REVERSING TYPE 2 DIABETES

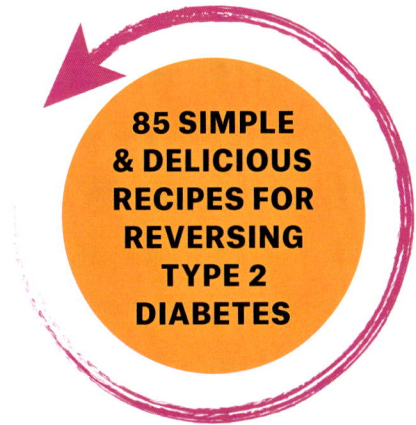

Life Without Diabetes
The Cookbook

Emma Porter

BASED ON THE 3-STEP PLAN BY PROFESSOR ROY TAYLOR

To my wonderful daughters, and enthusiastic taste testers, Florence and Clemmie.

First published in Great Britain in 2025 by
Short Books, an imprint of
Octopus Publishing Group Ltd
Carmelite House
50 Victoria Embankment
London EC4Y 0DZ
www.octopusbooks.co.uk

An Hachette UK Company
www.hachette.co.uk

The authorized representative in the EEA
is Hachette Ireland, 8 Castlecourt Centre,
Dublin 15, D15 XTP3, Ireland
(email: info@hbgi.ie)

Text copyright © Emma Porter 2025

Photography, design & layout copyright ©
Octopus Publishing Group 2025

Distributed in the US by Hachette Book
Group, 1290 Avenue of the Americas,
4th and 5th Floors, New York, NY 10104

Distributed in Canada by Canadian Manda
Group. 664 Annette St., Toronto,
Ontario, Canada M6S 2C8

Emma Porter asserts the moral right to be
identified as the author of this work.

ISBN 978 1 80419 224 5

A CIP catalogue record for this book is
available from the British Library.

Printed and bound in China.

10 9 8 7 6 5 4 3 2 1

Publisher: Jo Morrell
Senior Managing Editor: Sybella Stephens
Copy Editor: Lucy Bannell
Art Director: Nicky Collings
Photographer: Clare Winfield
Food Stylist: Kathy Kordalis
Props Stylist: Julie Patmore
Assistant Production Manager:
  Allison Gonsalves

Publisher's note
Nutritional calculations are based on single
servings using metric measures.

All reasonable care has been taken in
the preparation of this book but the
information it contains is not intended to
take the place of treatment by a qualified
medical practitioner.

Before making any changes in your health
regime, always consult a doctor. While
all the advice detailed in this book is
completely safe if done correctly, you must
seek professional advice if you are in any
doubt about any medical condition. Any
application of the ideas and information
contained in this book is at the reader's sole
discretion and risk.

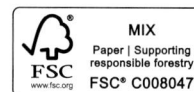

FSC
www.fsc.org

MIX
Paper | Supporting
responsible forestry
FSC® C008047

CONTENTS

FOREWORD

Food! What thoughts surface in your mind when you hear this word? Enjoyment? Exciting tastes? Variety? Family and/or friends? Health? These are all factors reflected in this book. And importantly, preparation time is short, for those with busy lives. This is a book of wonderful recipe ideas, all based on a highly effective programme for weight loss, which separates a rapid period of weight loss from the long-term challenge of avoiding weight regain. It is so successful that the NHS now recommend this for people who want to lose around 2½ stone (15kg) in weight in order to escape from type 2 diabetes. However, the health benefits of controlling weight go far beyond this, and the advice in this book is for anyone to take up – this book is for you if you want to enjoy life, and your wellbeing – and not just for people who have diabetes or pre-diabetes. It will make a huge difference to your health and how you feel from day-to-day if you have no medical problems, but have gained weight in adult life.

The standard health programme uses meal-replacement packets of soups or shakes, but the ingenuity of Emma's recipes in this book is that they offer people who wish to use real food the opportunity to seek better health via their kitchen. This is a science-based beacon of hope in a confused world of strident opinions about 'diets' and misleading adverts.

So, what happens to your food after it is swallowed? Where does it go inside you? My research at Newcastle University has been able to answer this question by using special MRI techniques to look inside the body and see what is happening. We now know why some people become unable to achieve healthy handling of food, resulting in heart trouble, type 2 diabetes and other health problems. The very practical outcome is that we have shown for the first time how and why type 2 diabetes can be reversed to normal, by weight loss followed by the long-term business of avoiding weight regain.

Back in 2008, I was faced with a big question. All our research pointed towards a simple hypothesis about what caused type 2 diabetes, but to test it rigorously my research volunteers would have to lose 2½ stone (15kg) in weight. How could this be done? Over several decades in my clinic, I had listened to many people describe their genuine problems of losing weight. Two major issues were regularly flagged up – the nagging hunger, and the burden of choosing what to eat and how much to eat at every mealtime – a bigger burden than most experts realise. Both problems were sorted by using a low calorie, rapid weight loss diet. On average, the volunteers lost the necessary weight in just 8 weeks.

Much to my surprise, our volunteers really liked the diet – largely because they rapidly felt more energetic. The most frequent comment was, 'I feel 10 years younger!' The elixir of youth was not a particular food, but rather shedding the weight that had crept on over many years. Yes, it was tough getting started on an 800-calorie diet, but within days the body had adapted with very positive results.

Putting all the research together there is a very simple message: your body has an amazing ability to deal with whatever food you eat, but it has no defence at all against eating more food than your body needs. That leads to a failure to properly deal with the incoming food. Some foods make you want to eat more of them and leave you feeling a bit peckish. Typically, ready meals, fast foods and many processed foods are designed to make you want to eat more. But why not have food which is enjoyable without a heavy calorie load? That is what this book is all about. Enjoy!

Professor Roy Taylor

INTRODUCTION

Welcome to a cookbook for your new lifestyle. These recipes will help improve your life if you have been diagnosed with diabetes. Type 1 diabetes is a lifelong condition that needs to be carefully controlled by insulin; type 2 diabetes can be vastly improved through diet, and the good news is that in many cases it can be reversed.

Dietary choices play a huge role in blood sugar management. I should know. I have type 1 diabetes and, for a time, experienced the symptoms of type 2 diabetes, too. I've spent more than a decade teaching thousands of people how they can reverse or better manage their type 2 diabetes and improve the control of their type 1 diabetes (alongside insulin) through food. Even though I know that I will always need insulin, I discovered through diet that I could improve the type 2 diabetes symptoms, and as a result I can better manage my type 1 diabetes. So, I get it: I get the struggle; I get how debilitating both mentally and physically all forms of diabetes can be. I understand how all-consuming and overwhelming weight gain can feel, and I empathize with the obsession for an instant fix. And I can honestly say, hand-on-heart, that this weight-loss process changed everything for me.

The recipes I have created for this book are based on Professor Roy Taylor's 3-step plan presented in his book *A Life Without Diabetes*, which you'll find out about in the next few pages. With this plan, I will guide you along a path to a healthier, happier and more confident you, where you can enjoy delicious food while controlling diabetes for life.

For me, it has been four years since I started the plan, and yes, life happens and stress happens (and I'm a stress-out-and-gain-weight kind of gal). So I have to manage it. I do that through going back to Step 1 of Professor Taylor's weight-management plan – using homemade shakes for a short time – when I need to. Step 2 is the gradual reintroduction of other foods, then Step 3 is the onward journey for the rest of your life, the best and forever part, accompanied by irresistible dishes that will both delight your palate and keep your condition stable.

I hope you will enjoy my wide and varied selection of recipes, and that they will entice and inspire you.

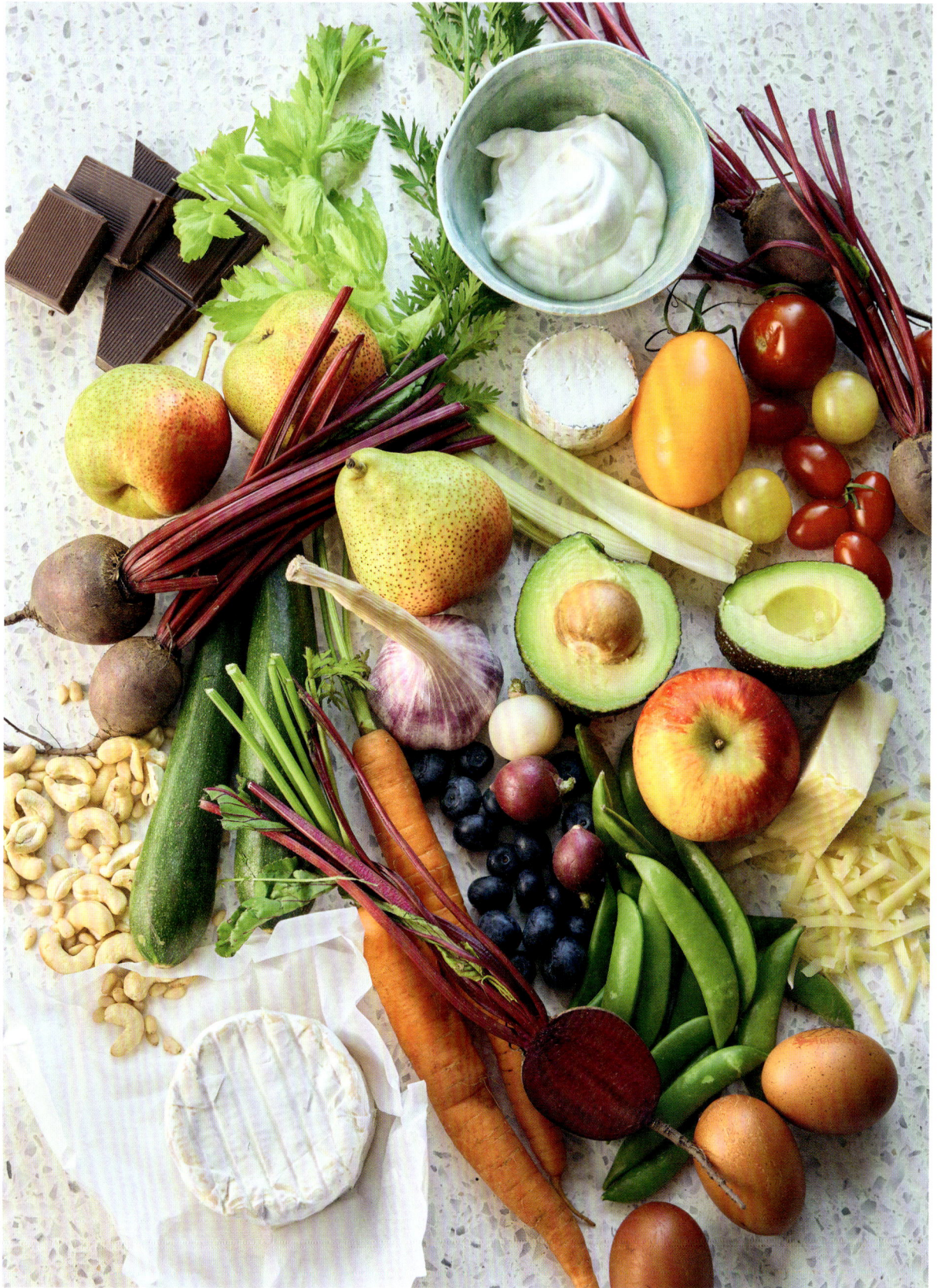

My journey

I was diagnosed with type 1 diabetes 20 years ago, as a teenager, which came as a shock to me and my family. For months, I had suffered with unquenchable thirst, the need to wee constantly, unexplained weight loss, muscle cramps, blurry vision and horrendous thrush.

At 17, I had that childhood air of invincibility and had never queried the rapidly increasing 'symptoms' as anything of any significance, and so they had continued for months before I finally went to the doctor at my boarding school, who performed a routine blood test. One evening after waking from a catatonic nine-hour 'nap', the headmaster tapped me on my shoulder and said I had to go to hospital, urgently.

At the hospital, a gaggle of nurses surrounded me firing questions: 'Can we prick your finger?' 'Can you do a urine sample?' 'Can I smell your breath?' 'Have you lost weight?' A nurse came in and shouted across the room, 'Where's the diabetic girl?' I looked around for her too, but then I realized the nurse was looking straight at me.

My blood sugar level was measured and found to be 56mmol (millimoles per litre). Normal levels tend to be 4–6mmol. The consultant later joked that this figure was the highest he'd seen and that I shouldn't have been able to stand. And that was my brutal introduction to life as a type 1 diabetic.

The first question I asked my consultant was whether I would put on weight as a result of taking insulin. 'Yes,' he said. 'Weight gain can be a typical side effect.' Another crushing blow, because having been a slightly overweight teenager, I had naively been thrilled with my effortless weight loss and the positive attention I was enjoying as a slim version of me. Little did I know how relentless and all-consuming my new condition would be and what a roller coaster I would be on for my weight.

And that was my somewhat brutal welcome to life as a type 1 diabetic. I hope your diagnosis has not been quite as dramatic! But I know, however you found out that you were diabetic, that it will have been a shock.

Taking control

Over the years, I must have tried pretty much every diet there is to control and manage my weight, while attempting to keep my blood sugars stable. It was like living a mission impossible, and my weight yo-yo-ed considerably. I followed general diabetes dietary advice but was still on a constant blood sugar roller coaster.

In 2013, my boyfriend and I became engaged while travelling in Indonesia. We decided we wanted to return to the same location for our wedding. Unfortunately, at this time, my health was deteriorating. I had been told I was showing early signs of diabetic retinopathy (eye disease), my weight was still difficult to control, my periods had stopped, I had constant brain fog, my mood was swinging like a pendulum and I was permanently exhausted. I decided that enough was enough and it was time to take charge of my health. I was going to get married on a beach and with a stable blood sugar level, and I was going to remember it... so I had a deadline.

I joined a gym and enrolled with a personal trainer, whose advice transformed my life. He introduced me to a lower carbohydrate (carb) diet. I focussed on eating real ingredients, cooking from scratch, no processed food and no grains. I started investigating low-carb diets online and followed the advice (people living with type 1 diabetes have to calculate their dose of insulin against the carbs in each meal, which is not the case for people with type 2 diabetes.)

Within a week I had slashed my insulin use by 60 per cent. I was bouncing out of bed before my alarm. In fact, I suddenly didn't even need the alarm. Over the weeks that followed, I lost several kilos in weight, my blood sugars fell to within the normal range, I didn't feel hungry and I felt more alert (no more brain fog!), more confident, happier and in control. 'In control' is something I had not ever felt before.

I started sharing the low-carb recipes I had created and pictures of what I was eating on a social media account and blog. People started to notice my weight loss and asked how I'd done it. My periods resumed and became regular. The only difference I had made to my life was to reduce the amount of carbs I was eating and quit the calorific, high-sugar, high-carb, low-fat lifestyle. By the time of our wedding, I felt and looked better than I ever had before. Not least because my blood sugars were in control.

For several years after getting married, I maintained excellent weight management and felt more in control of my diabetes than ever before. I gave birth to my first daughter in 2016. But then, shortly after my second daughter arrived, the unforeseen global pandemic occurred, completely turning my healthy lifestyle upside down.

A sudden realization

My second daughter was born on New Year's Eve in 2019. Only 12 weeks later, I was more or less the same size as before the pregnancy. My blood sugars were okay, but with the stresses of being a new mum, they were now navigating a new normal and my body was out of sync. As the months ticked by, my eldest daughter started school, but as we were in lockdown instead of going to school, she was being taught at our kitchen table through Zoom while I was juggling a nine-month-old.

I didn't really notice that I'd been gaining weight, and while at home I just kept wearing my stretchy and comfortable maternity leggings. It was only in 2021, when I wanted to start exercising again, that I realized just how much weight I had put on. Gyms were closed, so I contacted a friend who was a personal trainer and, following the rules, we trained in his garage gym with the door wide open. He implemented a weekly weigh-in, but, if anything, my weight was increasing. (My muscle mass was increasing, too, but that was the only positive.) No matter the number, I always closed my eyes when I was weighed. My brilliant trainer would write the number in his notebook and close it, so I was none the wiser to the truth.

Diet-wise, I felt I was progressing well. For a long time, I had followed a low-carb lifestyle because it worked for my blood sugars. It had previously helped me to lose weight by making it easier to decrease total food intake and stabilize my blood sugars. It kept my hba1c (a handy indicator of diabetic control over a three month period) in the non-diabetic range. However, there was definitely something wrong. My ankles had started to swell up and I was taking the most insulin I had ever taken.

It was weigh-in day. Even though I didn't feel any lighter, I thought the number must have dropped by now. I had been exercising a lot and eating my usual diet, so I asked what I weighed. I assumed I would have hit the high 80 kilos (around 176lb), maybe 90 kilos... but no. 'You're 104kg (229lb).' Silence.

I couldn't understand what I was doing wrong. My trainer suggested I go home and install an app on my phone and track my intake of macronutrients (macros) – protein, carbs and fat – for a few days. 'What rubbish,' I thought. 'I count my carbs, surely that's all I need to know?' Well, dear reader. I was wrong.

I went home and downloaded a macro-tracking app which produced a light-bulb moment. I realized that I had been consuming around 3,400 calories per day – almost 50 per cent more than I needed to sustain my body – and the majority of them were from salad! On the first day I measured my macros, I discovered a simple salad contained 900 calories, a lot of which was from olive oil. I hadn't just been drizzling or spraying it on, but glugging it on.

At this point, I knew I had to change things fast, so I decided to go on an 800-calorie-a-day shake diet. I created the smoothies and shakes at home in my kitchen – three different and delicious recipes a day – so I could keep a close eye on my carb and insulin intake.

My body had clearly been waiting a long time for this moment, because within eight weeks I had lost 30kg (66lb). It was a real eye-opener for me about how unnatural that excess weight must have been for my body. Once I had lost this weight and could both see and feel the results, I reaped the rewards. My clothes fitted; my blood sugars were in control; I had come off the added insulin resistance for type 2 diabetes medication; my insulin requirements reverted back to being 60 per cent lower than they had been; and I was finally eating the same foods I had enjoyed before starting my weight-loss journey. This was all achieved by being more mindful about portion sizes and understanding calories as well as carbs. I implemented some of the tips and tricks you will find throughout this book, such as using a reusable spray bottle for olive oil, being aware of the size of my plate… and understanding what 'dessertness' is! (See page 181 to find out for yourself.)

I now know that this weight was over and beyond my 'personal fat threshold', as Professor Roy Taylor so clearly explains in A Life Without Diabetes. *Although my life will never be without diabetes, it's very obvious now that my body had been struggling with a weight it could not maintain.*

For me, sticking to a low-carb diet is key to keeping my blood sugars more stable and my insulin intake low. Professor Taylor's 3-step eating regime prevents my weight from swinging from high to low, and it helps maintain my hormone levels, too. Being aware of calories, and reverting to a Step 1 deficit when I need to, helps me feel in greater control of my body.

Starting from scratch

When I left home and bought my first set of dinner plates, I hadn't realized just how enormous they were until a friend came over for dinner. She commented on their size, turned one of them over and read from the label on the base: 'charger plate'. I didn't even know what that was, but my friend explained we had been eating not from a dinner plate, but from a dinner-plate holder! My weight had been steadily increasing, but not for a second had I considered that it could be because I was filling my giant-sized dinner plate with food my body just did not need.

I grew up with an 'eat what's on your plate' mentality. I had also attended boarding school, where meals were fast, evenings were long and we always had somewhere to go – a club, a sports match or another lesson – so food was just fuel. We would all wolf down our dinner in the rush to get out. Over the years since, I have had to retrain myself to appreciate food and to eat mindfully rather than mindlessly.

Healthy food and lifestyle habits

I have found success by following rules, changing habits and focusing on sustainable practices that I can use in everyday life. This approach has not only led to my better physical health (sustained weight loss being one aspect of that), but also helped me to establish a positive relationship with food. This has resulted in me feeling well, keeping my weight stable and being able to enjoy sharing foods with family and friends. Here are some of the healthier food and lifestyle habits I have established for my long-term health, many of which are validated in Professor Taylor's 1-2-3 approach and which I hope will help you, too, gain success.

Tips for long-term health

- Use smaller-sized dinner plates to help manage your portion control.

- Use the size of your hands as a portion guide: a thumb for fat (butter, cheese and so on); a palm for protein (such as chicken breast or beef burger).

- Walking. The most underrated exercise, but from my perspective as someone living with diabetes, the most valuable. A brisk ten-minute walk can make a positive difference to both your mental and physical health. I realize that this advice from me is from a young, mobile person's perspective, and that it may not be possible for all.

- Stay hydrated and drink clear fluids throughout the day. I find that drinking a pint of cold water upon waking helps set me up for the day ahead. (If plain water doesn't appeal to you, see page 17.)

- Eat slowly and away from distractions such as television screens.

- Eat something sweet at the end of a meal rather than snacking in-between meals.

- The 3-step approach recommends not eating between meals. But, if you're struggling, select high-protein snack foods to keep you satisfied. Have a look at my Mackerel & Creamy Chive Dip, Perfect Soft-boiled 'Jammy' Eggs with Chilli & Almond Butter, Multiseed Crackers, or Greek yogurt: the sweet-toothed diabetic's best friend (see pages 69, 96, 178 and 181) for inspiration, but be disciplined with portion control.

- Do not eat straight out of a container: instead plate up, sit down and savour the flavours.

- Do not drink your calories. Many drinks – such as takeaway coffees and alcohol – contain added sugars and are calorie-dense. Read the labels on milks and dairy alternatives, as they all have different nutritional profiles.

- Opt for full-fat dairy products – butter, cheese, milk and yogurt – and eat them in small portions, rather than choosing low-fat dairy, which often contains additives and sugars.

- Prepare food from scratch whenever possible. This involves planning ahead, so try to get into that habit.

- Be aware of portion sizes and always read food labels to be aware of added ingredients.

- Shop online for food to resist temptation in the supermarket. Hidden salts and sugars are everywhere and supermarkets know exactly how to tempt you. They have two-for-the-price-of-one deals – note that you never find healthier options such as smoked salmon or extra virgin olive oil on offer – and they position their most-alluring snacks at the end of the aisles. Get wise to their tactics.

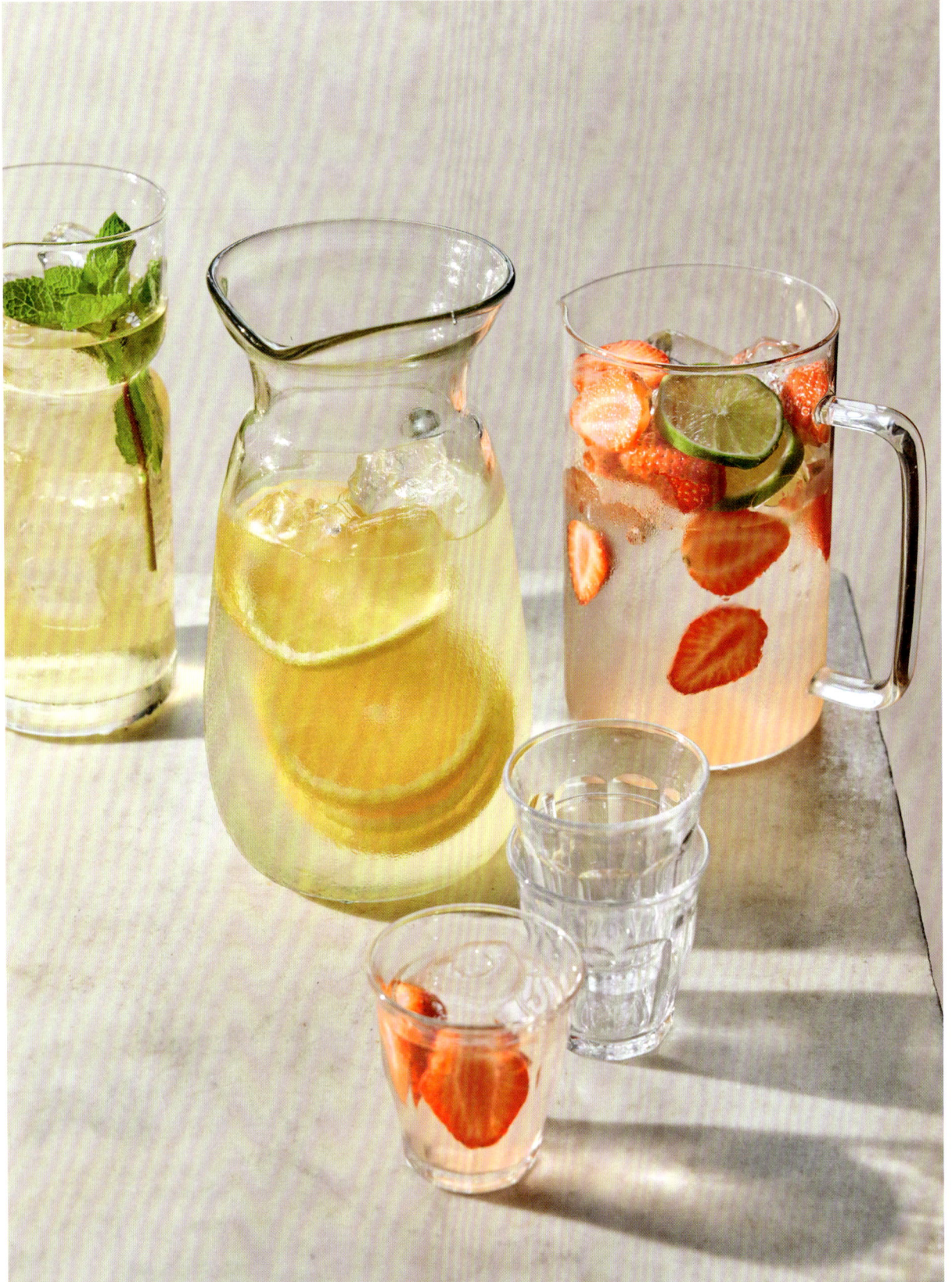

Hydration is key

If you are not a huge fan of water, you can flavour it to make it more appealing:

- Add the juice of 2 limes to 2 litres (2 quarts) water. Add sliced strawberries and lots of ice.

- Pop 6 peppermint teabags into a jug and pour in 7.5cm (3 inches) of boiling water. Once cooled, remove the teabags and add the mint-infused concentrate to a jug with 2 litres (2 quarts) cold water and lots of ice. Add mint leaves to serve.

- Fill a jug with 1 sliced orange and 2 litres (2 quarts) cold water. Leave to infuse for a few hours before serving with lots of ice.

I personally avoid ultra-processed sugar-free concentrates and cordials, as they can have a negative effect on my blood sugars. However, if you prefer sugar-free squash to the options above and they get you drinking more water, then hooray for hydration!

Cooking with fats

We know how versatile and health-friendly olive oil can be and it is important to reap its rewards, but it is also very calorie-dense, so be mindful of the amount you are using (as you might remember from my light-bulb moment, see page 13).

Buy yourself an empty reusable spray bottle. (Many ready-to-use spray bottles of oils and fats have added ingredients we just don't need, see page 18.) If you would rather buy a pre-filled spray, opt for one that contains only olive oil, without any additives.

Once you've filled your spray bottle with extra virgin olive oil, or light olive oil (see page 18 for the difference), you will be able to lightly coat pans, baking sheets or grills to prevent food from sticking to them during cooking or baking. A spray bottle will also add a lovely light dressing to a salad, while reducing the overall calorie and fat content.

Though decanting olive oil into a spray bottle does not guarantee reduced calories, it helps to control the amount you use, which in turn helps manage calorie intake. A spray of olive oil will measure about 15 kcal.

Understanding fats

Ultimately, the choice of oil or fat you cook with at any point depends on the cooking method you intend to use, your flavour preferences and desired health benefits.

Extra virgin olive oil
Best for creating dips and sauces, drizzling over salads or for cooking on medium or low heat, such as when sautéing vegetables.

Light olive oil
This has a milder flavour than extra virgin olive oil and can be used for frying, baking and grilling.

Olive oil
A versatile all-purpose olive oil, lighter flavoured than extra virgin olive oil and perfect for frying, roasting and everyday cooking. Great for dressings, marinades and baking, too.

Mixed spray olive oil
Many ready-filled olive oil spray bottles are composed of refined olive oil and extra virgin olive oils. Water, alcohol, emulsifiers, natural flavourings and thickeners can be added.

Coconut oil
Ideal for high-heat cooking such as frying and baking, and also used in vegan baking recipes for its distinct flavour and texture. Great in raw or non-baked desserts too. You can buy odourless coconut oil, which has all the benefits without the taste.

Avocado oil
This has a high smoke point, which makes it suitable for cooking methods such as frying and grilling, as well as for salad dressings and dips.

Butter
Adds richness and flavour and is commonly used in baking, sautéing and finishing sauces. Opt for unsalted butter (you can always add salt if you need to and this helps to moderate your salt intake).

Ghee
Similar to butter but with the milk solids removed. It has a higher smoke point than butter and is commonly used in Indian cooking for frying, sautéing and adding flavour to dishes.

Sesame oil
Used in Asian cuisine for stir-frying, sautéing and adding flavour to dishes, this adds a lovely nuttiness to salads and dips.

Equipment

I have tried to make the methods and equipment used as simple as possible in this book, but there are recipes where you will need certain gadgets. Here's a list of items I use in addition to standard kitchen utensils.

- High-powered blender, for soups and smoothies.

- Stick blender, great for blending soups straight in the pan.

- 450g (1lb) loaf tin for bread.

- 900g (2lb) loaf tin for cakes.

- Silicone baking mat: I cannot recommend these highly enough. They are nonstick, made from high-quality food-grade silicone and are available in several shapes and sizes to fit different baking sheets, cake tins and baking dishes, or they can also be cut to size. They are reusable and you don't need to grease them before placing food directly on top, saving the need to use butter or oils and thus reducing hidden calories. I have used the same mats for many years now. I love them as they are very easy to clean, especially compared to scrubbing a baking sheet with food baked on to it.

- Food processor: brilliant and versatile. I have had mine for more than a decade. It is super-sturdy and can easily chop, slice, grate and purée almost any food. I use it for many desserts, cauliflower 'rice' (see page 126) and dips.

- Mandolin: though not a necessity, this is fast and efficient at creating uniformly sliced vegetables. It is amazing for my Apple Layered Cake (see page 197).

- Spiralizer: I really recommend one of these, though it isn't a necessity as you can use a vegetable peeler to replicate items such as courgette 'noodles'. (see page 49).

Store cupboard and refrigerator

The key to making healthier food choices is in planning and preparation. I have to work hard on my mindset and maintaining healthy habits as best I can, and perhaps you do, too. Try not to leave planning and preparing until you feel 'hangry', as this only leads to mindless eating and / or food shopping.

Prepare your week's meal plan on a Sunday (see pages 202–4 for some examples for each step of the 1-2-3 plan). Write down the goals you want to achieve, which should be realistic so that you can stick to them. Prepare an online shop if necessary. Shopping online can really help prevent mid-aisle snacking, or accidentally demolishing a pack of biscuits in the car on the way home, singing along to the radio. (Of course, that is not something I have ever done…)

When you first start a new eating regime, you might open the kitchen cupboard and find a random mix of unsuitable ingredients, snacks and easy-to-munch-on treats. So one of your first tasks could be to remove those: look through your cupboards and remove any temptation. As we know, such 'treats' do not fill you up, they spike your blood sugars and they just leave you wanting more. Trust me, I have been there: normally at night, once the children are asleep, exhaustion is high, it is dark and rainy outside, and I find myself – in a trance – opening the snack cupboard of blood-sugar and weight-gain doom!

Quick-fix foods rarely ever fill the hunger void, so drinking a glass of water and distracting yourself for a while until you can source something more nutritious is always preferable. Try to have homemade options to hand or things like meats, cheeses, eggs, fruit, vegetable crudités, dips, Greek yogurt, nuts, seeds and dark chocolate (70 per cent cocoa solids).

In the 1-2-3 approach, eating between meals is not recommended. But let's be realistic: some of us have an urgent need for 'something' sometimes, so having some ready-made Multiseed Crackers with homemade dips and some crudités or some Lemon and Sesame Kale Crisps to hand (see pages 178 and 65) might help you win the war against grabbing a packet of something sugary or salty or calorific. I always keep my favourite type of apples in the refrigerator as a go-to snack, which I slice up and drizzle with a teaspoon of almond butter or peanut butter.

Many of us are actively trying to reduce the amount of ultra-processed food we are eating. By cooking with real food ingredients, you can take better control of what you are eating. If you are buying cans and packaged foods, take a look at the ingredients. Always read the labels and check the packaging for hidden additives, sugars, salts and artificial flavourings and sweeteners. Source the best food you can afford and opt for high-quality protein foods, especially eggs, meat and fish.

If you do shop in a supermarket rather than online, then take a shopping list and a bottle of water, eat before shopping and shop alone! Breaking old habits can be hard, but starting new ones can be refreshing and better for your long-term health goals. Walk around the supermarket with intent and purpose. Avoid the aisles you know will be too much of a temptation: bread and bakery, cereal, cakes, chocolates and sweets. It might seem hard the first few times, but the act of avoiding them will make you feel incentivized that you are prioritizing your health.

Store cupboard

These are essential ingredients and foods I use regularly, but it is only a guide and I hope it will inspire you and that you will enjoy adding your own items to the list.

Oils and fats

- Light olive oil
- Extra virgin olive oil
- Avocado oil
- Butter
- Coconut oil
- Ghee
- Sesame oil

Cans

- Canned tomatoes
- Canned coconut milk
- Canned oily fish: mackerel in olive oil, brine or water; sardines; salmon
- Canned chickpeas, cannellini beans and other pulses (fabulous for a quick meal such as my One-Pan Veggie Bean Brunch with Eggs, or Chickpea Dal see pages 106 and 129)

Other staples

- Apple cider vinegar
- Chickpea flour (also known as gram flour)
- Chocolate (at least 70 per cent cocoa solids)
- Coconut flour
- Eggs (opt for free-range)
- Gluten-free plain flour
- Ground almonds
- Ground flaxseed / linseed, and other milled seeds
- Harissa paste
- Jumbo oats
- Konjac noodles (also known as shirataki or skinny noodles)
- Miso paste
- Mixed whole seeds
- Pepper
- Sea salt flakes (for cooking and sprinkling over foods such as boiled eggs; avoid 'table salt')
- Soy sauce
- Stock cubes (vegetable and chicken)
- Sweetener: erythritol, stevia, xylitol (be wary, as xylitol is toxic for dogs)
- Tamari
- Vanilla pod or extract

Arrowroot

This deserves a little explanation, as this powder is an ingredient I have been using a lot in the last decade. It's an inexpensive starch for recipes such as pancakes, Yorkshire puddings and so on. It helps batters to bind and improves the consistency of certain foods. I really recommend it. You will find it in health food shops and the baking aisles of larger supermarkets, usually next to the baking powder. You only ever use a small amount. Cornflour is similar and more readily accessible, however, you need to use two-thirds more to get the same effect, which of course increases calories and carbs.

Spices and herbs

I will never forget opening my parents' herbs and spices drawer and finding a jar of ground cumin with an expiry date of 1990! Many ground spices have a shelf life of two or three years, whole spices usually a little more, so it is worth checking the packaging. Ground spices will lose their smell, colour and aroma over time. Combined with a small pinch of sea salt flakes, spices can really transform a dish. If you are buying blends of ground spices such as curry powder, have a look at the packaging and avoid those that contain additives, extra salt or sugar.

Dried herbs are a fabulous addition to your kitchen cupboards and many have a shelf life of a couple of years.

Here's a list of some of the spices and herbs I use regularly.

- Black pepper
- Cayenne pepper
- Chilli flakes
- Cinnamon
- Cumin (ground and seeds)
- Fennel seeds
- Garam masala
- Ginger
- Nutmeg
- Paprika
- Smoked paprika
- Turmeric
- Vanilla (pod)

- Basil
- Bay leaves
- Chives
- Coriander
- Dill
- Mint
- Oregano
- Parsley
- Rosemary
- Sage
- Tarragon
- Thyme

Freezer

My freezer staples include:

- Fruit: berries, cherries, mango and pineapple
- Herbs: to avoid waste, you can chop fresh herbs into ice-cube trays, add water to freeze and use at a later date.
- Frozen vegetables such as spinach, cauliflower rice, chopped pepper, diced onion (portion them up into food and freezer bags, ready to flash fry or add to things like curries and stews)
- Ice
- King prawns

Refrigerator

Effective and efficient food storage is essential and it's important to know how to stock your refrigerator properly to avoid temptation, allow easy access to the contents and to maintain hygiene. Once you have a neat and well-organized refrigerator, you will easily be able to reach all your ingredients and have less temptation to open the door and graze on the wrong foods. Ensure that foods are stored correctly to prevent any cross-contamination.

The bottom drawer of the refrigerator is ideal for fruit, herbs and vegetables. Remove any loose dirt and soil before storing vegetables. It is important to thoroughly wash all fruit, vegetables and salads that will be eaten raw, unless they have been pre-prepared and are specifically labelled 'ready to eat'.

The lowest shelf above the vegetable drawer is best for storing proteins such as fish, meat and chicken, as this is one of the coldest parts of the refrigerator. Ensure any meat and fish is wrapped and sealed.

Keep the middle shelf for dairy products such as cheese, butter, cream and yogurt.

The top shelf is for ready-to-eat foods and jars (sauerkraut, pickles, olives, garlic and ginger purées). They should be kept well away from any raw meats and harmful bacteria.

Dairy

Low-fat dairy products often contain added sugar or sweetener. Instead, opt for full-fat dairy when selecting your cheeses and yogurt, especially if you are also cooking for children.

Full-fat live Greek yogurt should only contain two ingredients: milk and bacteria. It is rich in protein and a good source of calcium. Please do check the packaging, as the list of added ingredients can be eye-opening. Low-fat yogurts invariably have extra ingredients, including sugar, which is added to make it more palatable after the removal of fat. If you opt for natural fat-free Greek yogurt, check the packaging to ensure there are no additives. Not all that is marked low-fat is low in calories! If you follow either a plant-based or vegan diet, select an alternative that you are happy with, such as natural unsweetened coconut yogurt. And if you haven't already done so, do try unsweetened kefir. This is pasteurized cow's milk fermented with live kefir cultures. High in protein, it provides a great base for a dressing: try adding lemon juice, chopped herbs and a sprinkling of flaky sea salt.

Sweeteners and sugars

We can all spot sources of sugar – cakes, biscuits, sweets and chocolates – but you might be surprised to hear that it lurks in so-called 'healthy' foods too. Many low-fat products, including yogurts, soups, high-protein bars, condiments, fruit juices, salad dressings, shop-bought coffees, smoothies and pasta sauces, are full of it. This makes foods addictive and all too easy to eat.

Many products prominently labelled 'healthy', 'gluten-free' or even 'sugar-free' in fact contain two or three different sugars. Sugar can be disguised under different names: corn sugar, dextrose, fructose, glucose, high-fructose glucose syrup, honey, maple syrup, agave syrup… Natural sugars such as honey, agave or maple syrup are often included to make products seem 'healthier', and though small amounts can make a palatable difference, many foods are saturated in the stuff, resulting in excess calories. *Sugar-free doesn't mean free of all sugars!* Sugar-free products are often still high in carbohydrates, which can be very confusing to the consumer and problematic if you are insulin-dependent with type 1 diabetes and end up underestimating the carb content.

As someone with type 1 diabetes, I know how impactful sugar is on my health, as I see how how high it can send my blood sugars. After years of developing recipes, I have tried many different types of sugars and sweeteners. Sweeteners are my preference, as they are often zero calorie, zero carb and have little to no impact on my blood sugars, while improving a food's palatability. The amount of sweetener, and the type you choose, depends on personal taste. Remember, with sweeteners: less is always more! Adding too much can ruin a dish. Some sweeteners can also cause stomach issues, so you might need to try a few different brands before finding one that works for you. Of course, you could just use sugar instead, but you will need to adjust the nutritional information accordingly, as the calories and carbs will both increase significantly.

My sweetener of choice is erythritol, readily available and sold in most large supermarkets, health food shops and online. I buy it in both white and brown granulated and powdered form and a little goes a long way. Erythritol is a sugar alcohol found in fruit, vegetables and fermented foods. It has zero calories and zero carbs. It is one of the sweeteners that is usually well tolerated, as 90 per cent of erythritol is absorbed by your digestive system and thus excreted in your urine. (There are a lot of alternative sweeteners out there, and it is up to you to choose what works best. My suggestions would be stevia, monk fruit and xylitol, but do note it is toxic for dogs.) Ultimately, the decision about whether to use sugar or sweetener – or neither – is yours, but being aware of where sugar is hidden will help you make informed health choices.

HOW TO USE THIS BOOK

You might be totally new to the Professor Taylor 1-2-3 approach, or perhaps looking for a variety of low-calorie meals. Whatever your reasons, this book is for you.

Though you can easily use this book on its own, I recommend strengthening your understanding of the 1-2-3 approach by reading Professor Taylor's book *A Life Without Diabetes*. Write down your weight-loss goals and some positive affirmations about why you want to achieve remission. How will I look when I lose weight? What will I be able to do? These notes can be really helpful if you start finding it difficult to continue. Share your goals with someone close to you, because during the first eight weeks you want to make life as simple as possible to prevent yourself from falling off the wagon. Below is a brief summary of the 1-2-3 plan.

Step 1

For eight weeks, you will be consuming three calorie-controlled smoothies, shakes or soups a day, with one plate of low-starch vegetables. If you choose to make the recipes from scratch, write down a list of ingredients you will need for the week. (See pages 202–4 for weekly meal plans.) Choose the recipes that you enjoy the most, so you have something to look forward to. Step 1 might feel a little restrictive to start with, but the recipes have been designed to taste delicious and make you feel full. Feeling hungry in the first 36 hours is normal, but after that the feeling fades as your body gets into fat-burning mode. If you find this step challenging, remember that recovering your health is so worthwhile.

Track your weight weekly and write it down. Seeing the positive news from the scales will incentivize you to persist with Step 1 until you achieve your target weight. The amount of weight loss you need to achieve may be considerable and is best viewed as you would view an essential surgical operation: a short term restriction on everyday life, but a huge long-term benefit. If you have type 2 diabetes, the plan is designed to reverse the underlying cause and to restore your health. Step 1 is designed to take about 8 weeks, but if you need a little longer that is fine.

Step 2

Once you have achieved your target weight loss, move on to Step 2 by replacing one of your shakes or soups for lunch or dinner with a low-calorie meal. When you feel ready, replace a second meal, then finally introduce all breakfasts, lunches and dinners as meals. At first you should aim to consume approximately 400 calories for lunch and 400–500 calories for dinner (refer to the calorie counts for each recipe). How long this takes is entirely down to you as an individual. Step 2 should not be rushed, as you are setting the scene for life-long eating. Just replace the next meal when you feel ready – usually after 1–2 weeks for each. If you find your weight is creeping back up at any time, simply reintroduce Step 1 to get back on track.

In summary, this is what happens in Step 2 over the course of 3–6 weeks:

First: add a low-calorie meal to replace a 200 calorie soup or shake (you should be consuming 2 soups/shakes plus 1 solid meal per day).

Next: add in a second meal (you will be consuming 1 shake or soup plus 2 solid meals per day)

Finally: Add a third larger meal – you are now ready for a long-term pattern of eating, and Step 3.

Step 3

This is the maintenance phase, to keep your weight and blood sugars stable for life. You need to be aware of the correct portion size you need to avoid weight regain, as well as the calorie content of your food. Using all the tools in this book – awareness of portion control, labelling and shopping tips – arm yourself with the ability to prevent any relapse into type 2 diabetes and better control your type 1 diabetes.

If you fall off the wagon, just start again when you are ready. This often happens when you experience stress in your life. Don't beat yourself up, as that is never healthy. Remember, at any stage, you can always revert to Step 1 for a reset.

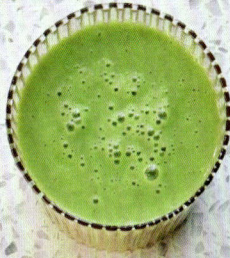

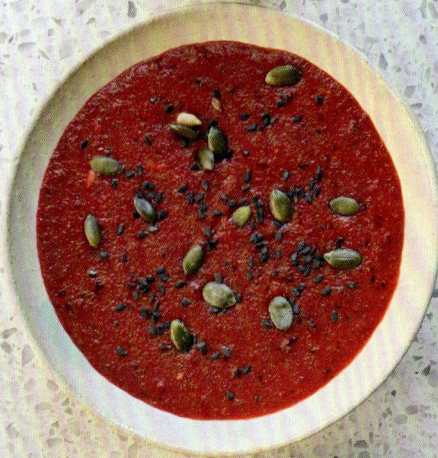

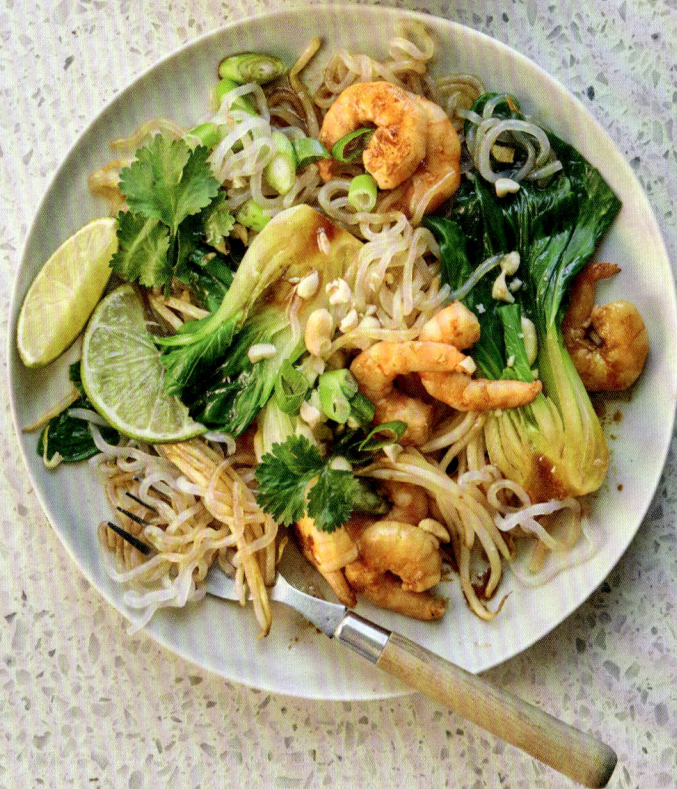

STEP

ONE

WELCOME TO STEP 1.

This is the rapid weight-loss phase, in which you switch your normal meals for three calorie-controlled meal replacement shakes, smoothies or soups, plus one low-starch vegetable plate per day. You will be eating around 800 calories a day, usually for a period of eight weeks. But ideally, Step 1 ends when you have reached your target weight.

There are of course commercially available packets of liquid formula diet that you can choose to buy instead of making your own which are quick and convenient. Although these might take away a lot of the burden of decisions about what and how much to eat, I think it's much better – and tastier – to make your own!

The recipes that follow for homemade shakes, smoothies and soups are bright and vibrant, created from scratch using wholesome everyday, real food ingredients. My low-starch vegetable plates are designed to provide you with fibre, as well as give you something to chew – these are intended to be eaten in addition to the shakes, smoothies and soups which can be enjoyed either for lunch or as an evening meal.

While you are in Step 1, you will need to prepare for the week ahead, to ensure you have the correct ingredients. Kitchen scales and a measuring jug are important to ensure accurate measurements.

Your daily intake of sugar from my homemade smoothies and shakes will be much less than the body makes for itself in a day, and under these weight-loss conditions it does not push up blood sugar for those living with type 2 diabetes.

Full nutritional calculations including calories, net carbs, fibre, protein and fat for a single portion are provided alongside each recipe. Calculations are based on the recipe stated, and do not include any serving suggestions or side dishes.

With it all laid out like this, preparing a daily 800-calorie diet becomes achievable, making life as straightforward as possible for you.

While a balanced diet is the ideal way to obtain essential vitamins and minerals, it can be challenging to ensure all your nutritional needs are fully met, especially during steps 1 and 2. To address this, I suggest taking a multivitamin to help fill any nutritional gaps and offer assurance.

How to achieve perfect smoothies and shakes

To keep your smoothies low in calories but tasty, cool and creamy, follow these tips:

Fruit

Frozen fruit is readily available, nutritionally dense and will thicken a smoothie without the need for much ice, if any at all. Alternatively, you can use fresh fruit and add ice. To learn more about frozen berries, see page 33.

Liquid

To keep calories on the lower side, my recipes tend to use unsweetened almond milk. Please ensure you buy an unsweetened variety and always keep an eye on the packaging for added ingredients. Other good choices are water, coconut water or other low-calorie unsweetened nut milks, and Greek yogurt and kefir are brilliant, too. If you would prefer to use dairy milk, you can keep the calories down by using skimmed milk.

Ice

Have ice cubes to hand in the freezer when making smoothies using fresh fruit or vegetables. It acts as a thickener, giving smoothies a creamy, frothy and indulgent texture.

Sweetener

A sweetener such as powdered erythritol contains no calories, and powdered sweeteners blend into smoothies without leaving any granulated remains. Add sweetener only after tasting the finished smoothie to check you really need it, as some can be overpowering. Start by adding 5g or 1 teaspoon at a time and give it a good stir. Taste, then add more if necessary.

Ingredient order

Putting smoothie ingredients into your blender in the correct order will place less stress on the motor and help achieve a smooth consistency.

1. liquid or yogurt
2. soft fruit or veg
3. greens
4. any nut butters, extra seeds or powders (except sweeteners)
5. ice or frozen fruit
6. sweetener (add after tasting)

Fibre

The smoothie recipes that follow in this chapter all contain a healthy dose of fibre, but feel free to scatter over more for added texture. For an added fibre boost, try:

2 teaspoons (10g / $\frac{1}{4}$oz) chia seeds (20 kcal)

1 tablespoon flaxseeds / linseeds (20 kcal)

70g (2$\frac{1}{2}$oz) berries (such as raspberries, strawberries or blueberries) (20 kcal)

If the texture of your smoothie is thicker or coarser than usual, you might prefer to enjoy it as a smoothie bowl, eaten with a spoon, instead of in a glass.

Protein

This is the most filling macronutrient. Eating a sufficient amount helps you feel less hungry and you'll consume fewer calories. However, not all protein sources are equal and the exact amount each of us needs is totally individual. As a rough guide, the recomended average intake for a woman is 45g (1½oz) per day, and 55g (2oz) per day for a man – bear this in mind when selecting which meals to have each day. Protein seems to have become a real buzz word and 'high protein' is emblazoned on the packaging of health-focused foods, from bars and yogurts to shakes and soups. However, despite the health-focussed messaging, these products are often full of added sugars and salts and are high in carbs. Though they tend to be more expensive than non-labelled high-protein products, they will rarely achieve like-for-like nutrition.

These days, many smoothie recipes include protein powder. A typical serving of protein powder will add 15–30g (½–1oz) protein to a smoothie. There are many brands on the market, so work out which is best for you: some are vegan, some are fast-release for a quick fix, and others are slow-release and best taken at bedtime. Whatever you choose, always consider the type of protein it contains as well as its flavour, texture and affordability, and go for brands that are minimally processed and without added sugars, salts and sweeteners.

For my smoothie recipes, I use unsweetened, flavourless whey protein. You could also use plant-based pea protein powder or skimmed milk powder.

Other ingredients to add protein to smoothies:

Full-fat natural Greek yogurt
(100g / 3½oz portion = 6g protein + 50 kcal)

Fat-free cottage cheese
(75g / 2½oz portion = 8g protein + 46 kcal)

Unsweetened kefir
(100ml / 3½fl oz portion = 3.5g protein + 59 kcal)

Unsweetened soy milk (100ml / 3½fl oz portion
= 3.3g protein + 33 kcal)

Unsweetened, additive-free nut butter, such as almond or peanut butter
(15g / ½oz serving = 3.5g protein + 87 kcal)

Unsalted peanuts
(25g / 1oz serving = 6g protein + 146 kcal)

Hemp seed
(20g / ¾oz serving = 7g protein + 113 kcal)

Flaxseeds / linseeds
(20g / ¾oz serving = 5g protein + 100 kcal)

Chia seeds
(15g / ½oz serving = 3.3g protein + 62 kcal)

Egg white
(2 egg whites = 7.6g protein + 30 kcal)*

Tofu
(70g / 2½oz serving = 11.6g protein + 100 kcal)

*Note: egg whites for eating raw should be from eggs that have the British Lion stamp, as these will be free from salmonella.

Frozen berries

If you're living with diabetes, these are a superhero food. Not only are they convenient, nutritious and versatile, but they are also low-calorie and low-carb, so they're brilliant to incorporate into your diet. You will find lots of recipes in this book that use frozen berries, so grab a bag next time you are in the supermarket.

Nutrient retention
Frozen berries are picked at peak ripeness and quickly frozen, which helps lock in their nutrients. They retain their vitamins, minerals and antioxidants even after being frozen.

Convenience
They are available year-round and can be stored for an extended period to use whenever you need them. They also eliminate the need for washing and cutting fresh fruit, saving time in meal preparation. You'll see in these recipes, especially in Step 1 and Step 2, that I've tried to reduce your kitchen prepping time to reduce the temptation to snack on other foods while you're in the room.

Cost-effective
Depending on the season and your location, frozen berries can be more affordable than fresh, especially if you're buying out-of-season fruit.

Versatility
Frozen berries can be used in smoothies, desserts, baked goods and toppings for yogurts, among many other ways (check the index for a full list). They add a burst of flavour and vibrant colour to any recipe.

Texture
They often have a slightly firmer texture than fresh fruit, which can be desirable in certain recipes, such as smoothies.

THE ULTIMATE GREEN SMOOTHIE

SERVES

1

250ml (9fl oz) coconut water, plus more if needed

juice of ½ lime

40g (1½oz) avocado, peeled and pitted

2 handfuls of spinach

1 small pear, chopped

1 tablespoon unsweetened flavourless whey protein powder

4–5 ice cubes

NET CARBS	27G
FIBRE	5.4G
PROTEIN	7.7G
FAT	7.5G
KCAL	221

PREP TIME

LESS THAN 5 MINS

No, this doesn't contain wheatgrass, kale or spirulina, but it is gloriously green, smooth and creamy, filling and subtly sweet. A delicious and nutritious smoothie, packed full of goodness. You could enjoy this as a smoothie bowl with a sprinkle of chia seeds for added crunch and fibre.

1 Place the coconut water, lime juice, avocado, spinach, pear, protein powder and ice in a smoothie maker (I use a high-powered blender).

2 Blend until smooth, adding a little more coconut water if you would like the texture to be thinner.

3 Serve immediately.

RECIPE TIP

If you have any smoothie leftover, keep it in the refrigerator and consume within 24 hours, or pour into ice-cube moulds and store in the freezer. You can add the frozen cubes to future smoothies for an extra dose of goodness.

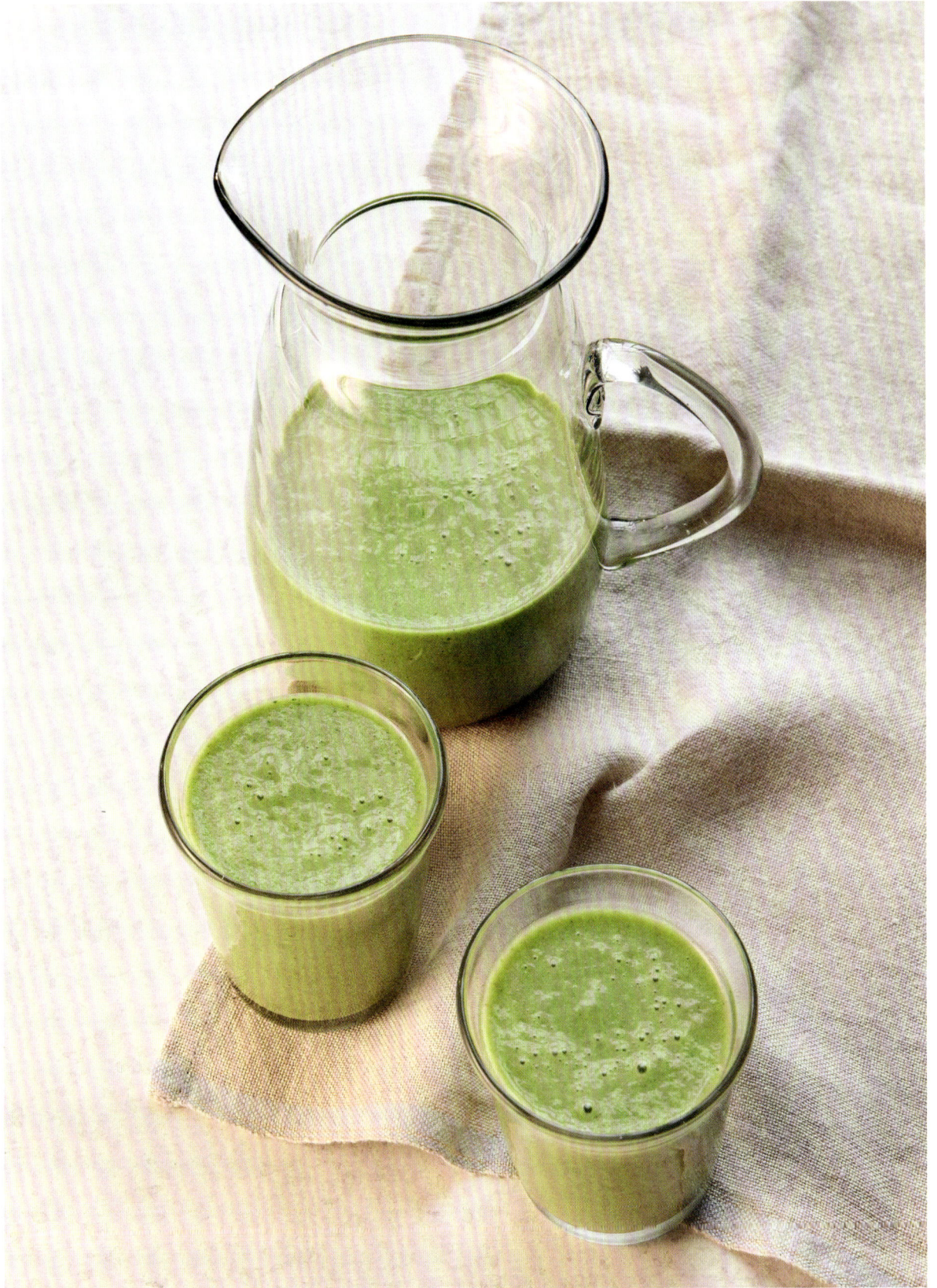

BLUEBERRY AND ALMOND BUTTER SMOOTHIE

SERVES
1

250ml (9fl oz) skimmed milk, or
  unsweetened almond milk (see
  recipe introduction), plus more if
  needed

50g (1¾oz) fresh blueberries

15g (½oz) 100 per cent almond butter

1 tablespoon unsweetened flavourless
  whey protein powder (optional,
  if using almond milk, see recipe
  introduction)

50g (1¾oz) frozen blueberries

NET CARBS	23G
FIBRE	4.7G
PROTEIN	20G
FAT	9.1G
KCAL	200

PREP TIME
LESS THAN 5 MINS

A quick and simple creamy smoothie that has the perfect balance
of energy, vitamins and fibre. There is absolutely no need for a
sweetener here, as it is sweet enough. If you are using skimmed milk,
this will provide you with an adequate amount of protein. However,
if you are using almond milk this is actually very low in protein, so
you will need to add a serving of protein powder.

1 Place all the ingredients in a smoothie maker (I use a high-powered
   blender) and blitz until smooth and creamy. Remember to add them
   in the correct order: liquid, fresh fruit, nut butter, then powder, if using,
   and finally frozen fruit. Add more milk if you would like a thinner
   consistency.

2 Serve immediately.

RECIPE TIP

Frozen blueberries are cheaper than fresh and brilliant for
smoothies, as they add creaminess and chill the drink, but
you can use all fresh blueberries instead, if that's what you
have, and blend the smoothie with a little ice.

CHERRY AND CHOCOLATE SMOOTHIE

SERVES
1

200ml (7fl oz) skimmed milk, or unsweetened almond milk, plus more if needed

60ml (4 tablespoons) low-fat coconut milk

1 tablespoon cocoa powder

1 tablespoon powdered sweetener

20g (¾oz) unsweetened flavourless whey protein powder (optional, if using almond milk)

80g (2¾oz) frozen cherries

NET CARBS	22G
FIBRE	3.5G
PROTEIN	28G
FAT	6.7G
KCAL	265

PREP TIME
LESS THAN 5 MINS

If you like chocolate, this is the perfect combination: both chocolatey *and* sweet from the cherries. I buy frozen cherries, available all year round and good value.

1 Place all the ingredients in a smoothie maker (I use a high-powered blender) and blitz until smooth and creamy. Remember to add them in the correct order: liquids, powders then frozen fruit. Add more milk if you would like a thinner consistency.

2 Serve immediately.

RECIPE TIP During Step 1 (see page 30), it is important to keep calories low, so skimmed milk or almond milk are preferable.

STRAWBERRY SHORTCAKE SHAKE

SERVES

1

200ml (7fl oz) skimmed milk, or unsweetened almond milk, plus more if needed

1 teaspoon sugar-free vanilla extract

120g (4¼oz) ripe strawberries, the sweeter the better

15g (½oz) 100 per cent cashew nut butter or 100 per cent almond butter

powdered sweetener, to taste

2 tablespoons unsweetened flavourless whey protein powder (optional, if using almond milk)

4–5 ice cubes

NET CARBS	25G
FIBRE	5G
PROTEIN	21G
FAT	8.6G
KCAL	253

PREP TIME

LESS THAN 5 MINS

This delicious shake tastes decadent, buttery and indulgent. I have suggested making a single serving, as it is important to be especially mindful of portion sizes in Step 1.

1 Place all the ingredients in a smoothie maker (I use a high-powered blender) and blitz until smooth and creamy. Remember to add them in the correct order: liquid, fresh fruit, nut butter, powdered sweetener to taste, the protein powder (if using), then ice. Add more milk if you would like a thinner consistency and more powdered sweetener if you like.

2 Serve immediately.

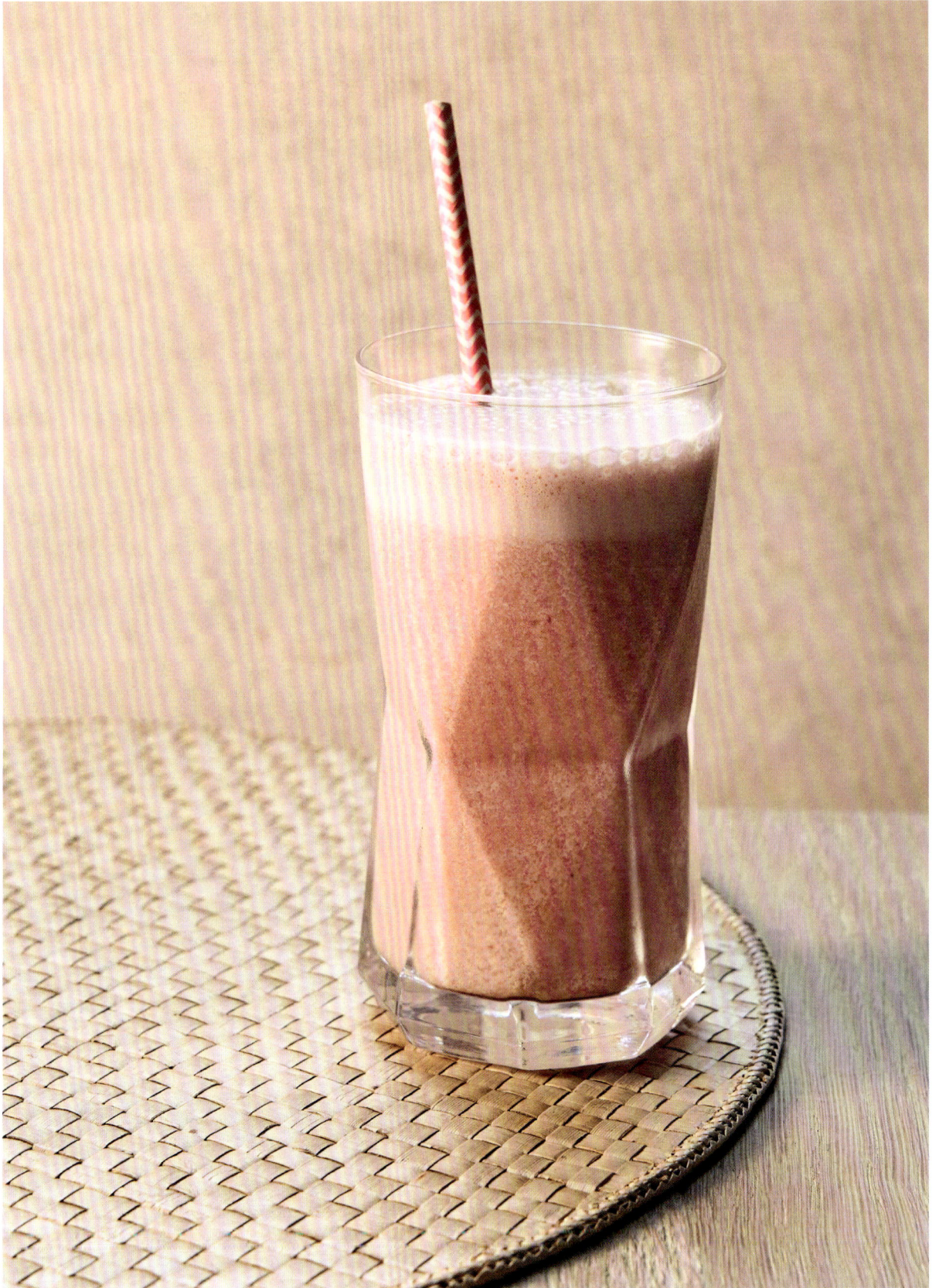

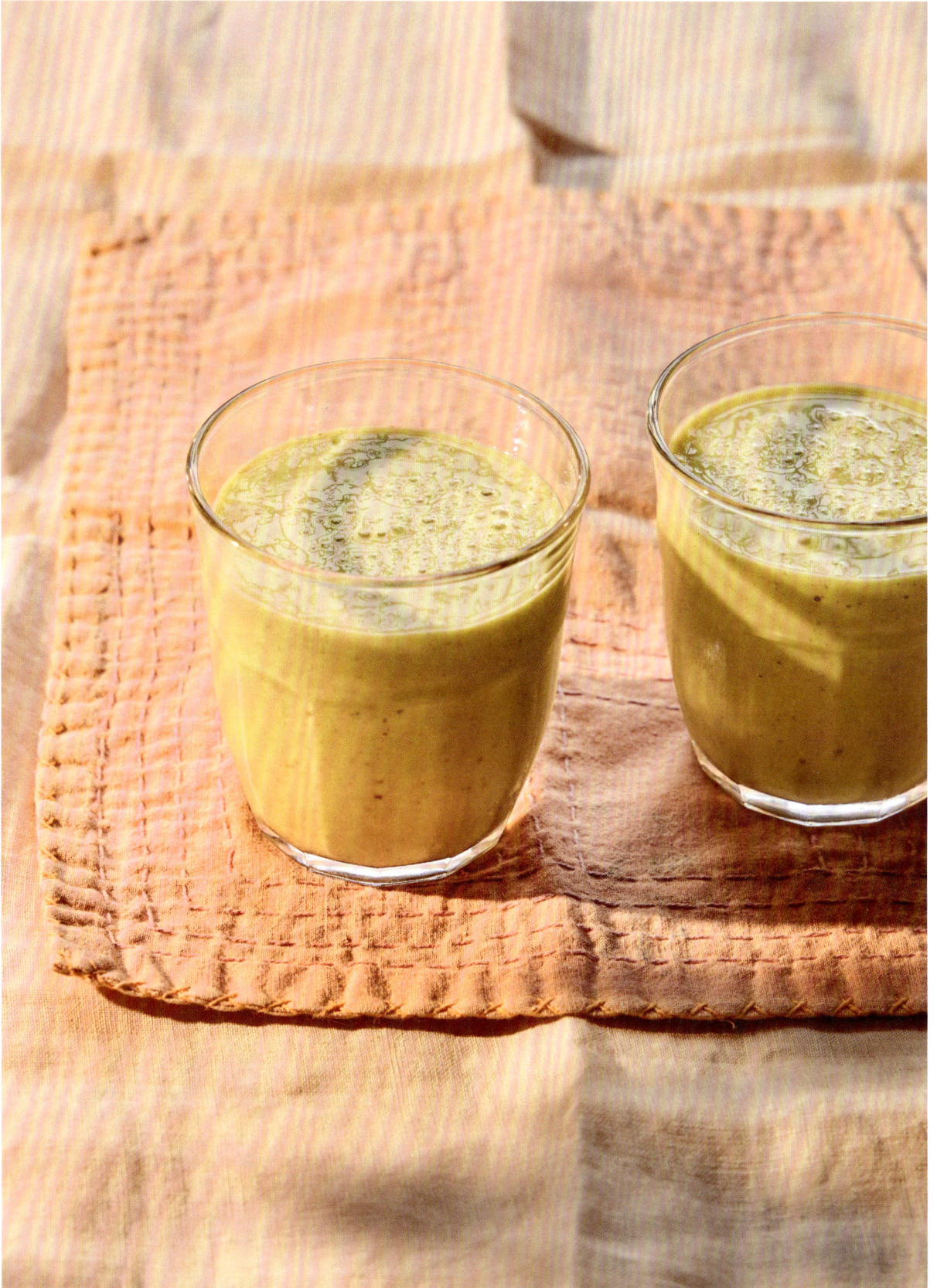

TOTALLY TROPICAL SMOOTHIE

SERVES
1

PREP TIME
5 MINS

260ml (9fl oz) skimmed milk, or unsweetened almond milk, plus more if needed

30g (2 tablespoons) low-fat coconut milk or fat-free Greek yogurt

handful of spinach leaves

1 teaspoon ground flaxseeds / linseeds, or ground chia seeds

½ teaspoon powdered sweetener (optional)

1 tablespoon unsweetened flavourless whey protein powder (optional, if using almond milk)

90g (3¼oz) frozen mango or pineapple chunks

Perfect for sunny days, or to brighten up a dark dreary one! When mangos are on offer, buy them, cut the flesh into little cubes and pop them into the freezer in 100g (3½oz) portions, ready for smoothies. It makes preparation quicker and easier and works out cheaper, too.

1 Place all the ingredients in a smoothie maker (I use a high-powered blender) and blitz until smooth and creamy. Remember to add them in the correct order: liquid, greens, seeds and powders, if using, then finally frozen fruit. Add more milk if you would like a thinner consistency.

2 Serve immediately.

NET CARBS	25G
FIBRE	2.7G
PROTEIN	16G
FAT	4.9G
KCAL	213

RECIPE TIP
Why are the flaxseeds or chia seeds important? Because both types of seed provide a boost of fibre and also thicken a smoothie to make it more filling. Leave the smoothie to stand for 5 minutes after preparing it, and it will thicken as the seeds soak up the liquid.

FROZEN BERRY, KEFIR AND VANILLA SMOOTHIE

PERFECT SMOOTHIES AND SHAKES

SERVES
1

PREP TIME
5 MINS

200ml (7fl oz) skimmed milk, or
   unsweetened almond milk

100ml (3½fl oz) kefir

50g (1¾oz) fat-free Greek yogurt

2 teaspoons sugar-free vanilla extract

100g (3½oz) frozen mixed berries
   (I opt for mixed bags of strawberries,
   raspberries and blueberries)

15g (½oz) powdered sweetener,
   or to taste

NET CARBS	21G
FIBRE	3.6G
PROTEIN	19G
FAT	2.8G
KCAL	192

A gut-boosting, creamy smoothie that provides a good dose of protein, making it a nutritious and satisfying drink. As well as being good for those living with diabetes, children love this shake and it's ideal to give to them after a dose of antibiotics or during the winter, when their immune systems are a little low.

1 Place the milk, kefir, Greek yogurt and vanilla extract in a smoothie maker (I use a high-powered blender), then add the frozen berries. Blend until smooth and creamy. If the smoothie is too thick, you can add a little water to reach your desired consistency.

2 Taste the smoothie and add sweetener if needed. Pour into a glass and enjoy immediately.

RECIPE TIP

I suggest buying packs of frozen berries. Be wary of frozen other fruit such as grapes, banana, mango and pineapple, as these are higher in carbs and will cause a glucose spike.

KALE GLOW SMOOTHIE

SERVES
1

PREP TIME
5 MINS

240ml (8¾fl oz) skimmed milk, or
unsweetened almond milk

60g (2¼oz) spinach

50g (1¾oz) kale

20g (¾oz) unsweetened flavourless
whey protein powder

80g (2¾oz) frozen mango

4 ice cubes

powdered sweetener, to taste
(optional)

NET CARBS	22G
FIBRE	3.9G
PROTEIN	30G
FAT	2.6G
KCAL	241

This has a wonderful colour and texture, a subtle sweetness and is very filling too. Smoothies are often sweetened with dates and banana and sometimes have items such as oat milk and oats in them too. Type 1 diabetics like me have to actively avoid such combinations, but we can with this recipe, which is the perfect balance of vegetables and a little fruit.

1 Place the milk, spinach, kale, whey protein, frozen mango and ice cubes in a smoothie maker (I use a high-powered blender. Blend until smooth and creamy. If the smoothie is too thick, you can add a little water to reach your desired consistency.

2 Taste the smoothie and add sweetener if needed. Pour into a glass and enjoy immediately.

WATERCRESS, LEEK AND PEA SOUP

SERVES
4

PREP TIME
5 MINS

COOK TIME
20 MINS

1 tablespoon olive oil

1 tablespoon unsalted butter

340g (12oz) leeks, chopped

250g (9oz) onion, chopped

2 garlic cloves, crushed and chopped

900ml (1½ pints) vegetable stock, or chicken stock, made with a stock cube if you like

80g (2¾oz) watercress

250g (9oz) frozen peas

80g (2¾oz) Greek yogurt

sea salt flakes and freshly ground black pepper

PER SERVING	
NET CARBS	17G
FIBRE	7.5G
PROTEIN	7.6G
FAT	9.8G
KCAL	201

This reminds me of my childhood, as my mum used to make watercress soup and it was a favourite meal for me and my brother. Mum's was thickened with potato and served with a giant slice of hand-cut white bread smothered in butter. I wouldn't eat that with it these days, of course, but the beautiful vibrant green colour more than makes up for it!

1 Heat the oil and butter in a large saucepan and fry the leeks and onion until translucent and soft. Add the garlic and continue to cook until fragrant and softened.

2 Pour in the stock and bring to the boil. Add the watercress and cook just until wilted, then tip in the peas. Return to the boil, then reduce the heat and simmer for 10 minutes. You want to keep the soup vibrant and green, so be careful not to overcook it.

3 Using a stick blender, blend until smooth.

4 Spoon in the Greek yogurt and a pinch of salt and pepper. Mix together well, set over a medium heat and bring up to a bubble.

5 Serve immediately, or allow to fully cool, then place in an airtight container in the refrigerator and eat within 3 days, or freeze for up to 3 months. If freezing, defrost overnight, then return to the boil before serving.

RECIPE TIP
Keep a tablespoon of the cooked peas and a few watercress leaves to one side and use them to garnish, along with a swirl of extra yogurt and a twist of black pepper.

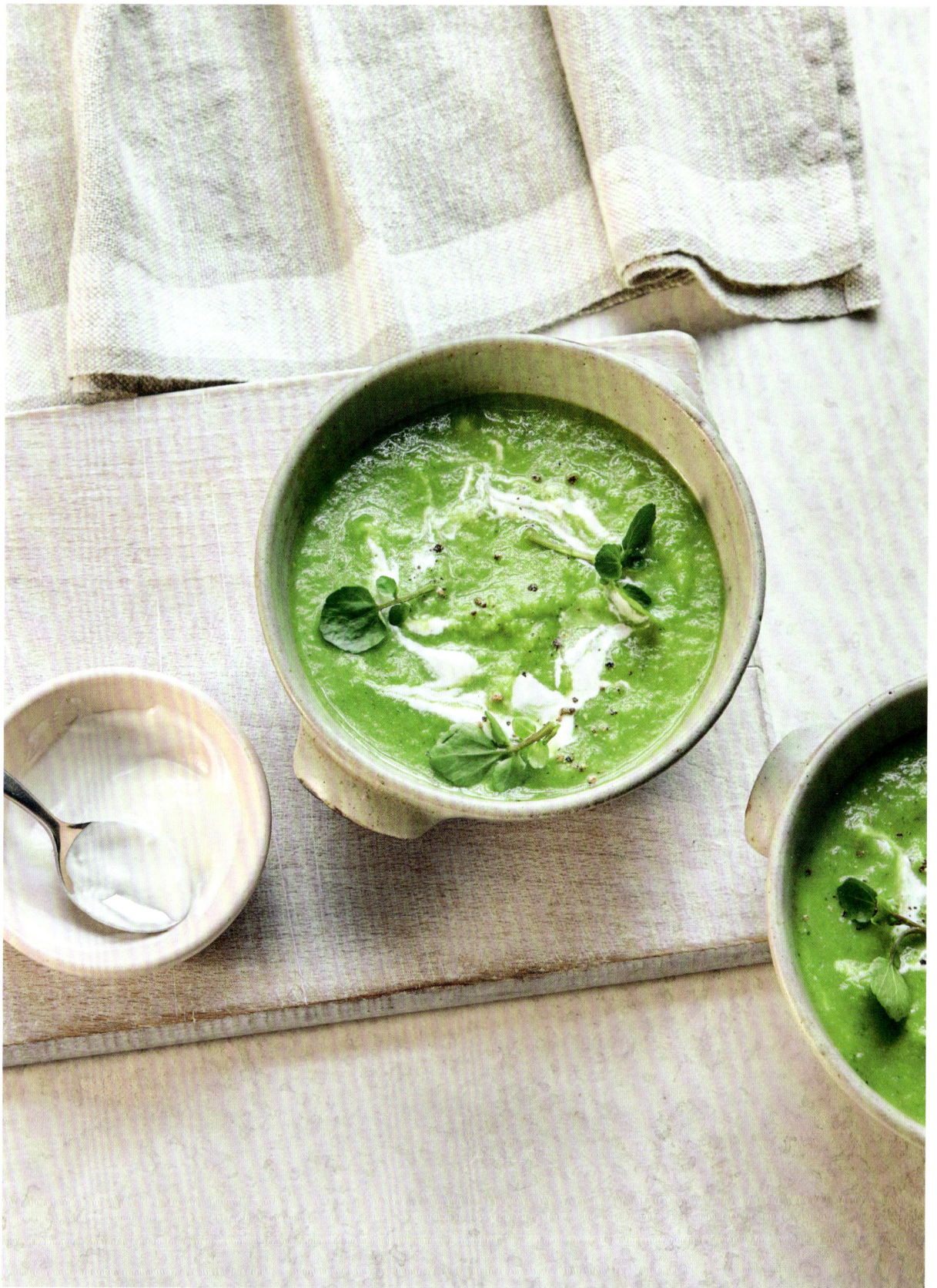

ALMOND AND CELERIAC SOUP

SERVES
4

PREP TIME
10 MINS

COOK TIME
40 MINS

1 teaspoon olive oil

1 onion, chopped

2 garlic cloves, chopped

2.5cm (1 inch) cube of fresh root ginger, chopped

100g (3½oz) ground almonds, ground cashew nuts, or ground flaxseeds / linseeds

600ml (1 pint) vegetable stock, made with a stock cube if you like

300g (10½oz) prepared celeriac, chopped

sea salt flakes and freshly ground black pepper

PER SERVING	
NET CARBS	7.3G
FIBRE	6.2G
PROTEIN	7.2G
FAT	17G
KCAL	223

My favourite one-pot effortless soup: creamy, decadent, filling and nutritious, it has been tweaked and refined over twenty years.
I first showcased it to a cooking class via Zoom during the Covid pandemic; to this day, the soup receives regular messages of praise!
Try garnishing it with some roasted shallot and a few toasted flaked almonds, or simply some finely chopped chives.

1 Heat a little olive oil in a large saucepan and fry the onion, garlic and ginger until the onion has caramelized and become translucent. Add the ground almonds and stir well.

2 Pour in the stock and bring to the boil. Add the celeriac, cover with the lid and reduce the temperature to a simmer. Cook for 30 minutes, checking it every few minutes and stirring if necessary. If the liquid is quickly disappearing, use your judgement and pour in a little more water.

3 Turn off the heat and test the celeriac with the point of a knife to make sure it is tender.

4 Purée with a stick blender until completely smooth. Taste and season with salt and pepper, then serve with another generous twist of pepper.

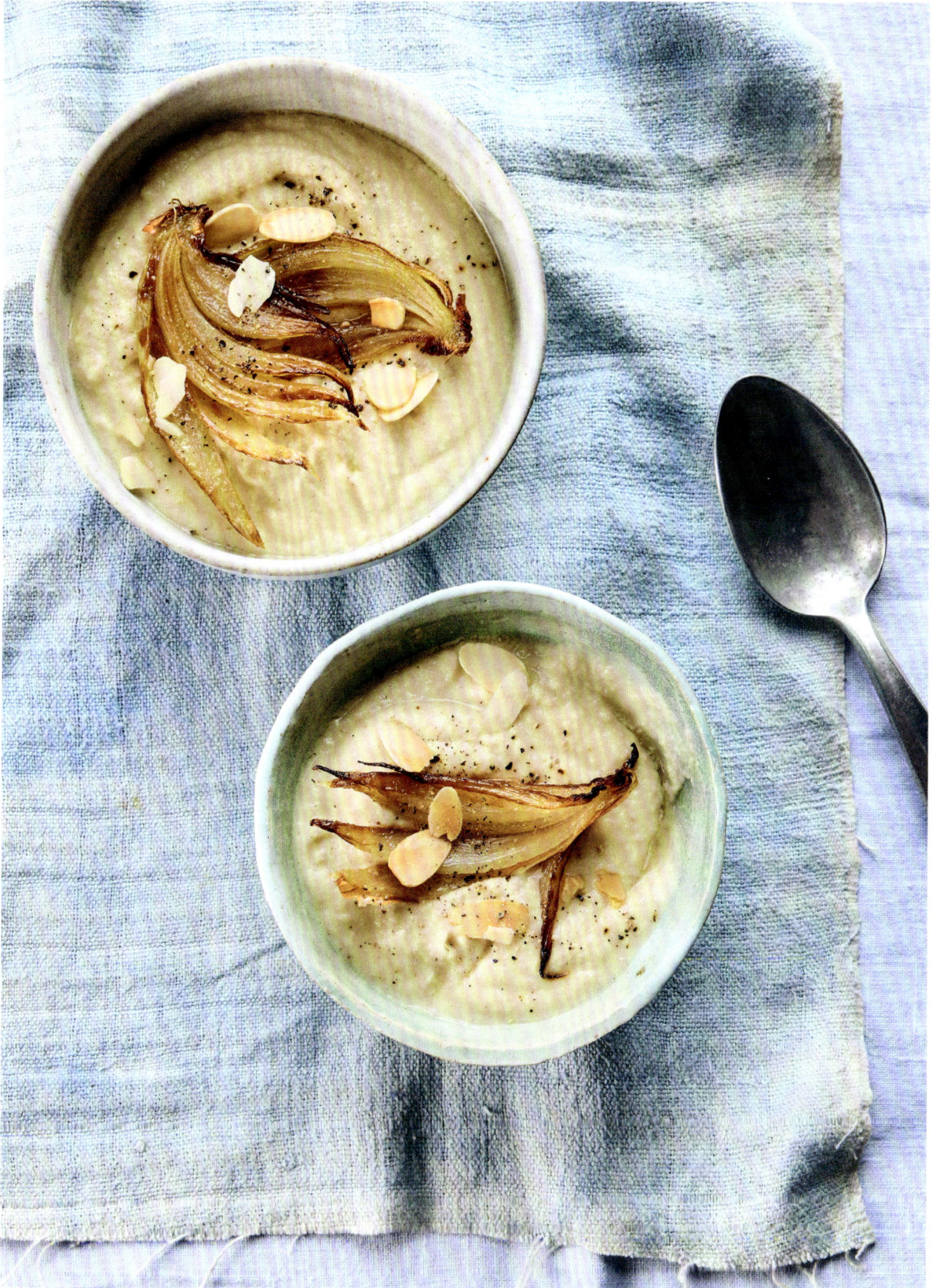

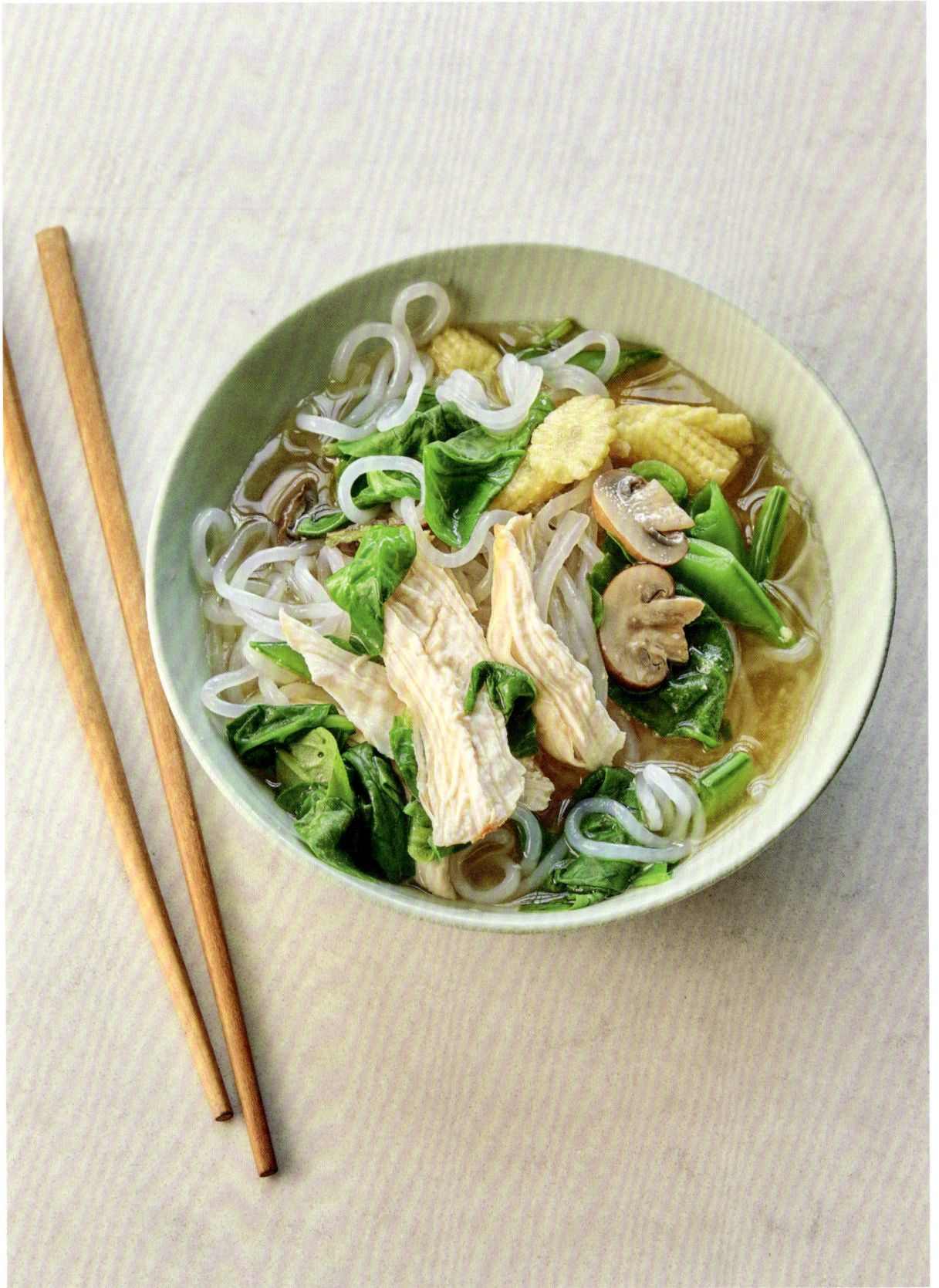

CHICKEN AND MISO NOODLE SOUP

SERVES
1

PREP TIME
LESS THAN
5 MINS

COOK TIME
5 MINS

200ml (7fl oz) water

50g (1¾oz) spinach leaves,
or pea shoots

50g (1¾oz) sliced stir-fry vegetables

20g (¾oz) miso paste from a jar or
sachet

125g (4½oz) konjac noodles or
courgette 'noodles'

60g (2¼oz) cooked skinless boneless
chicken, shredded or thinly sliced

NET CARBS	5.6G
FIBRE	2.6G
PROTEIN	24G
FAT	3.8G
KCAL	156

This recipe requires so little effort that you'll hardly believe it! It's a really convenient, super-tasty dish which is filling, low in calories and full of fibre. Depending on what I have in the cupboard, I either combine it with courgette 'noodles' (see page 58) or konjac noodles (also called shirataki, see page 142), as these noodles contain only 15 calories per serving, no carbs and are also very high in fibre, making them extremely filling. The miso adds taste and saltiness, the chicken contains all the protein you need and the low-starch veg provides added nourishment and nutrients. Use a bag of stir-fry vegetables to make things even quicker.

1 Bring the water to the boil in a saucepan.

2 Add the spinach or pea shoots, stir-fry vegetables and miso paste, then return to the boil. Once the spinach has wilted, add the konjac noodles or courgette 'noodles' and chicken and stir them through.

3 Carefully pour into a warmed bowl and serve.

SOUPS

RECIPE TIP If using courgette noodles (spiralized courgette), use 1 large courgette (approximately 160g/5¾oz each) per person.

ROASTED TOMATO AND RED PEPPER SOUP

SERVES
4

PREP TIME
10 MINS

COOK TIME
30 MINS

800g (1lb 12oz) ripe red tomatoes, halved

200g (7oz) courgette, chopped

2 red peppers, deseeded and roughly chopped

1 red onion, chopped

2 garlic cloves, unpeeled

2 tablespoons olive oil

300ml (½ pint) chicken stock, or vegetable stock, made with a stock cube if you like

thyme leaves or basil, to garnish

sea salt flakes and freshly ground black pepper

PER SERVING	
NET CARBS	14G
FIBRE	4.4G
PROTEIN	3G
FAT	7.1G
KCAL	149

Bright, vibrant and thoroughly delicious. You can add some chilli flakes for an extra kick, if you like.

1 Preheat the oven to 190°C (375°F), Gas Mark 5.

2 Place the tomatoes, courgette, peppers, onion and garlic in a roasting tray. Drizzle with 1 tablespoon of the oil and season with salt and pepper. Roast for 25 minutes, shaking the tray occasionally, until the vegetables are tender and fragrant.

3 Carefully remove the tray from the oven and allow the vegetables to cool for a few minutes.

4 Place the roasted vegetables in a deep saucepan with the remaining 1 tablespoon olive oil and the stock. Bring to the boil, then remove from the heat.

5 Blitz the soup with a stick blender until smooth. (Or you can use a blender.) Season to taste, and, if the soup is too thick, add a little water until it is the desired consistency.

6 Reheat in the pan, then serve garnished with some fresh herbs such as thyme or basil, and a twist of black pepper.

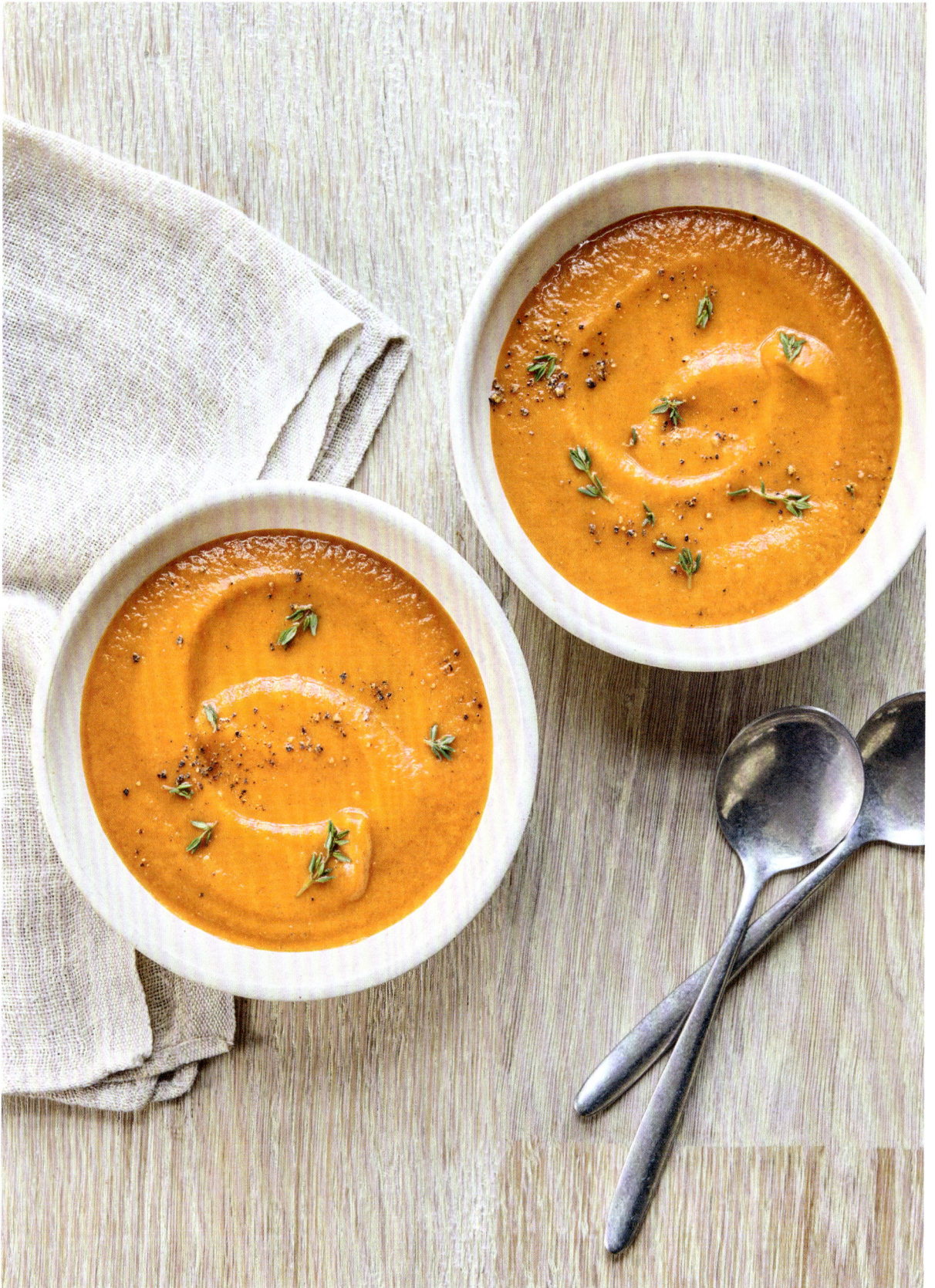

CREAM OF ASPARAGUS SOUP

SERVES
4

PREP TIME
5 MINS

COOK TIME
25 MINS

olive oil

180g (6oz) leeks, chopped

350g (12oz) asparagus spears, chopped

700ml (1¼ pints) vegetable stock,
   made with a stock cube if you like

200ml (7fl oz) coconut milk

sea salt flakes and cracked
   black pepper

chopped chives, to serve

PER SERVING	
NET CARBS	6.3G
FIBRE	3G
PROTEIN	4.5G
FAT	9.9G
KCAL	138

Asparagus is not only low in fat and calories – at just 20 calories per 100g / 3½oz – but it is also high in fibre and low in carbs too. Despite all that, it is rich in flavour and a beautiful creamy green colour.
It makes for a perfectly balanced nutritious soup for Step 1, or a fabulous lunch alongside some protein in Step 2.

1 Heat a little oil in a deep saucepan and cook the leeks, without allowing them to colour, for 2 minutes.

2 Add the asparagus and cook for a further 5 minutes or until starting to soften but not brown.

3 Pour in the stock and bring to the boil, then reduce the heat and simmer for 15 minutes.

4 Add the coconut milk, a pinch of salt and 1 teaspoon pepper, then blend with a stick blender until smooth, or carefully pour into a food processor and blend. Taste the soup and adjust the seasoning, if needed.

5 Serve scattered with chopped chives.

CREAMY MUSHROOM SOUP

SERVES
4

PREP TIME
10 MINS

COOK TIME
25 MINUTES

2 tablespoons olive oil

150g (5½oz) onion, chopped

2 garlic cloves, finely chopped

400g (14oz) mushrooms, finely sliced

650ml (1 pint 1¾fl oz) vegetable stock, or chicken stock, made with a stock cube if you like

¼ teaspoon grated nutmeg

2 tablespoons Greek yogurt

150ml (¼ pint) coconut milk

sea salt and cracked black pepper

chopped chives, to serve (optional)

PER SERVING	
NET CARBS	8.3G
FIBRE	1.3G
PROTEIN	4.8G
FAT	15G
KCAL	187

A decadent-tasting soup using very simple ingredients which are easy to find. My whole family love this, and it's quick and simple to make.

1 Heat the olive oil in a large saucepan over a high heat. Add the onion and sweat it for about 3 minutes or until softened and golden. Then add the garlic and mushrooms and fry for a further 3–4 minutes until the mushrooms are soft.

2 Pour in the stock, bring to the boil, then reduce the heat and simmer for 15 minutes.

3 Stir in the nutmeg, Greek yogurt and coconut milk and cook for a further 2 minutes.

4 Remove from the heat and allow to cool for a few minutes. Carefully pour the soup mixture into a blender and blend to a purée, or use a stick blender in the saucepan.

5 Return the soup to the pan, season to taste and reheat when ready to serve scattered with a sprinkle of chives, if you like.

SOUPS

BEETROOT, COCONUT AND GARLIC SOUP

SERVES
4

PREP TIME
15 MINS

COOK TIME
50 MINUTES

1 teaspoon coconut oil

1 red onion, sliced

2 large garlic cloves, sliced

2 teaspoons paprika

2 teaspoons ground cumin

600g (1lb 5oz) beetroot, peeled and cut into 5mm (¼ inch) cubes

600ml (1 pint) chicken stock, or vegetable stock, made with a stock cube if you like

400ml (14fl oz) can of low-fat coconut milk

sea salt flakes and freshly ground black pepper

PER SERVING	
NET CARBS	16G
FIBRE	5.1G
PROTEIN	4.5G
FAT	9.1G
KCAL	175

This warming, vibrant and flavour-packed velvety soup combines the earthy depth and richness of beetroot with the warmth of garlic and creaminess of coconut. If you are seeking a way to boost your protein intake, consider adding a touch of Greek yogurt, or a sprinkle of toasted nuts, which also add a satisfying crunch.

1 Melt the coconut oil in a deep saucepan over a high heat. Fry the onion until translucent. Add the garlic and fry until it is soft and golden brown, but don't allow it to burn. Add the paprika and cumin, then reduce the heat and stir to coat the onion with them.

2 Add the beetroot and stir to fully coat the cubes in the mixture, then fry for a further 3 minutes.

3 Pour in the stock and season with salt and pepper. Bring to the boil for a few minutes, then reduce the heat to a simmer and cook for around 40 minutes, or until the beetroot is fork-tender. (If you are using pre-cooked beetroot, you will only need to simmer it for 10 minutes.)

4 Blend the soup until smooth with a stick blender.

5 Return the pan to a low heat, add the coconut milk, then serve. Alternatively, leave until cold, then keep it in an airtight container in the refrigerator for up to 5 days, or freeze for up to 3 months – the flavours will improve the longer you leave it. To serve, fully defrost and reheat to boiling.

RECIPE TIP Use roasted or pre-cooked beetroot (drain before using) to make life quicker! If you want to roast the beetroot yourself, which is tastier, see page 71. Serve with a few mixed seeds on top if you like, but bare in mind this will increase the calories.

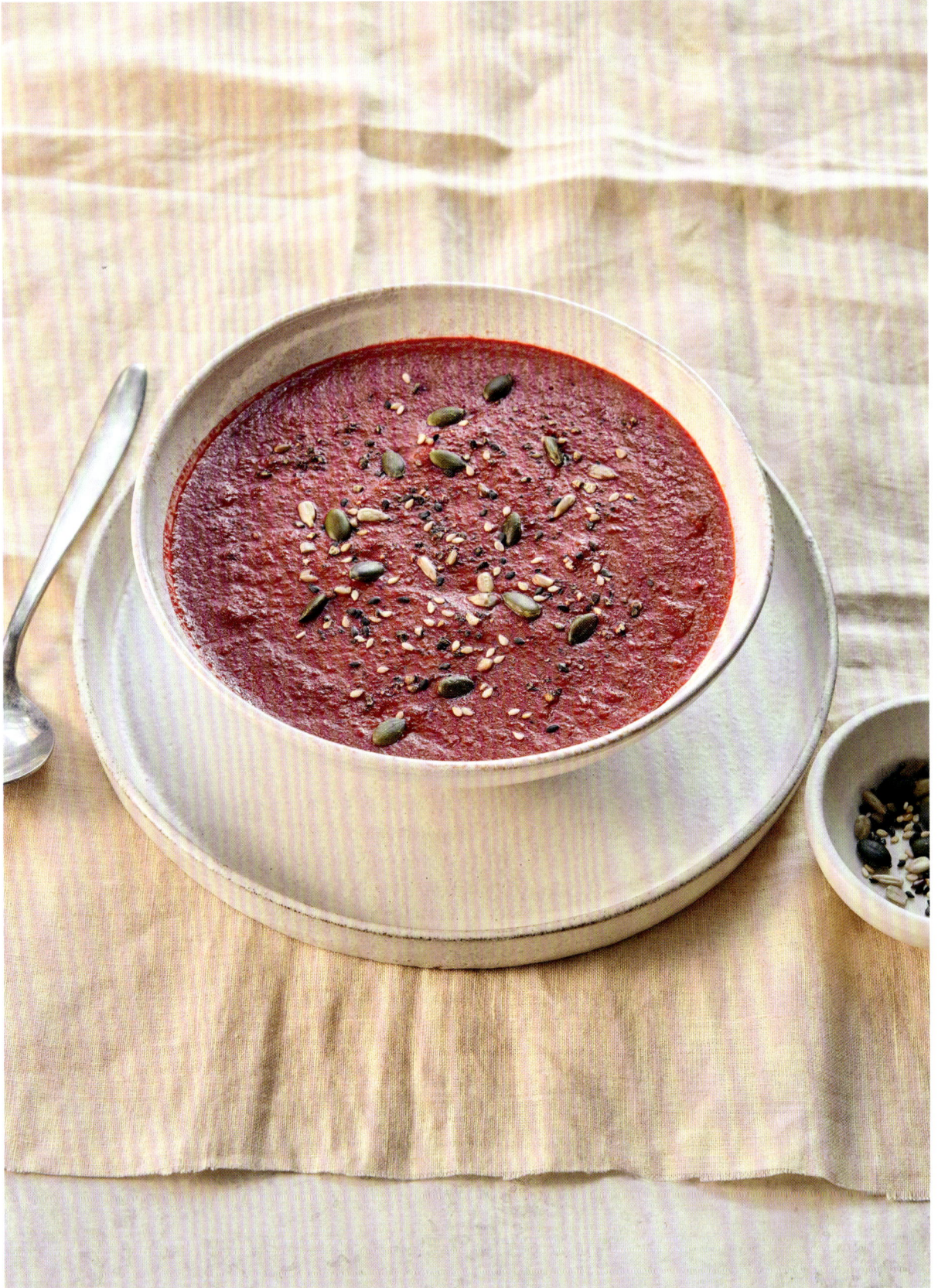

PICKLED CUCUMBER AND CELERY
WITH GARLIC AND GINGER

SERVES

3

1 cucumber, peeled

1 celery stalk, trimmed and finely sliced

1 tablespoon rice vinegar, or apple cider vinegar

1 teaspoon powdered sweetener

1 tablespoon low-salt soy sauce

1 teaspoon finely chopped, finely grated or puréed fresh root ginger

1 teaspoon garlic purée, or to taste

sesame seeds and a few coriander leaves, to garnish (optional)

PER SERVING	
NET CARBS	3.8G
FIBRE	1.8G
PROTEIN	2.4G
FAT	1.2G
KCAL	39

PREP TIME

10 MINUTES,
PLUS CHILLING TIME

A tangy, taste-tantalizing sensation that complements most dishes. It is perfect as part of a meal when you are in Steps 2 or 3, but also delicious on its own during Step 1 to provide a satisfying crunch.

1 Halve the cucumber lengthways, then scoop out the seeds with a teaspoon and discard or compost them. Cut the cucumber into slices and put them into a container (don't use metal, which might react with the vinegar). Add the celery.

2 Place the vinegar, sweetener, soy sauce, ginger and garlic in a separate small bowl and mix well together, then pour it over the cucumber and celery and mix thoroughly.

3 Cover and chill for at least 30 minutes until required. You can stir the veg occasionally to ensure they stay coated in the vinegar mix. Serve scattered with a pinch of sesame seeds and a few coriander leaves if you like. Eat within 3 days.

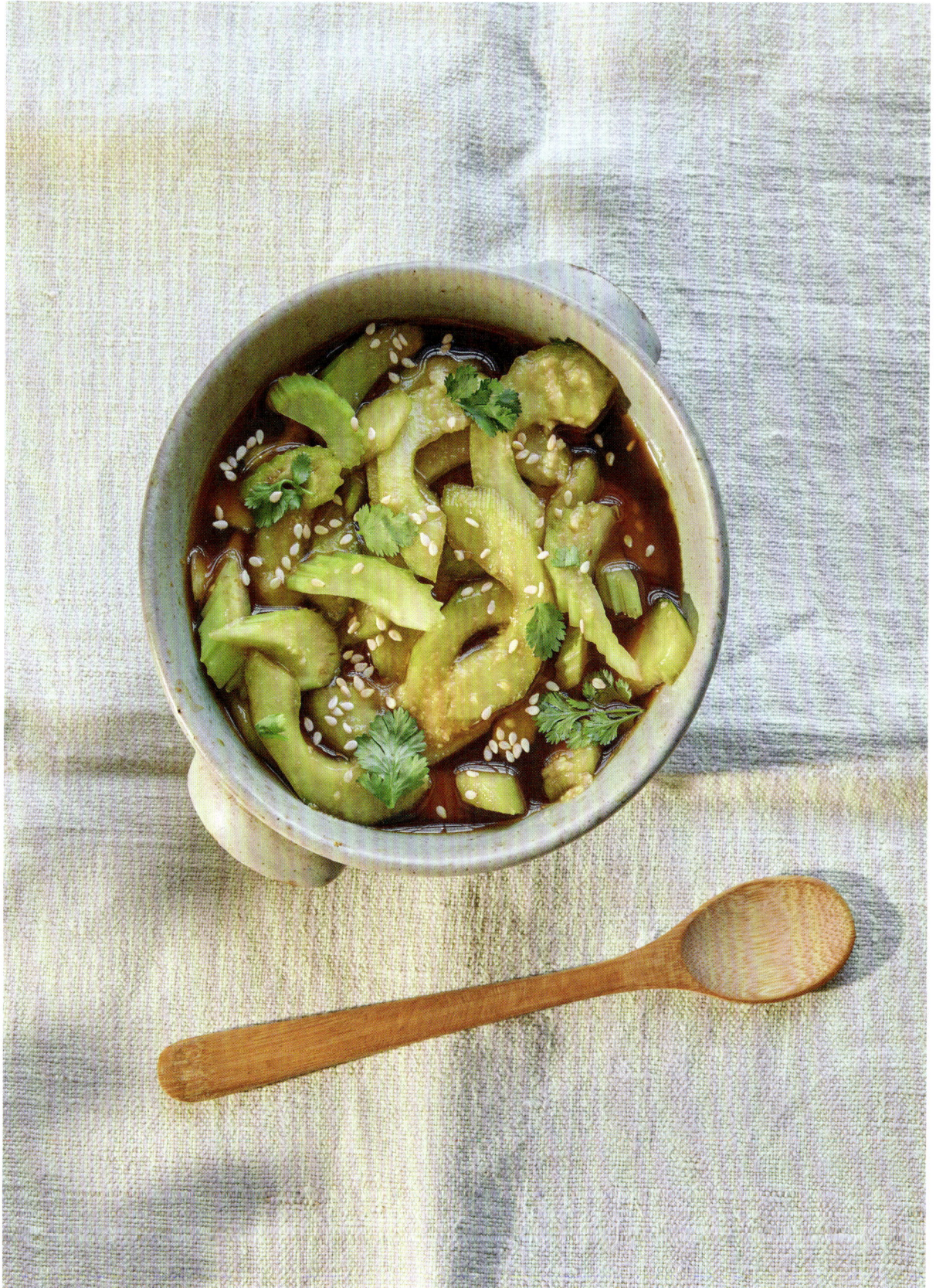

TANGY COURGETTE 'NOODLES'
WITH CORIANDER, CHILLI, SOY AND SESAME

SERVES
2

PREP TIME
10 MINS

COOK TIME
2 MINS

300g (10½oz) courgette, spiralized into 'noodles' (see below)

1 teaspoon sesame oil

15g (½oz) fresh coriander leaves, chopped

½ small red chilli, finely sliced

15g (½oz) low-salt soy sauce

5g (18oz) sesame seeds

PER SERVING	
NET CARBS	4.4G
FIBRE	2.2G
PROTEIN	3.8G
FAT	6.8G
KCAL	98

I first served this dish on a wellness retreat alongside chicken satay skewers, and it was the talk of the night! The guests were pleasantly surprised at how a simple courgette could be transformed into tempting, taste-packed 'noodles'. It is light, flavoursome and low in calories, making it a healthy side dish to enjoy with a smoothie during Step 1, or serve it as a large salad with a portion of protein during Steps 2 or 3.

1 Place the courgette 'noodles' in a large mixing bowl.

2 Put the sesame oil, coriander, chilli and soy sauce into a separate bowl and mix. Pour this mixture over the courgette and toss together to ensure everything is coated.

3 Dry-fry the sesame seeds in a frying pan over a medium heat until fragrant. Scatter them over the dish, plate up and enjoy!

HOW TO MAKE COURGETTE 'NOODLES'

Curly, long, vibrant and fresh, veggie 'noodles' are an excellent natural substitute for pasta. A spiralizer is a great kitchen utensil – it's one of my favourites – but you can use a vegetable peeler instead. To make vegetable 'noodles' with a peeler, thinly peel down the length of the courgette from top to bottom (this also works with similar vegetables such as cucumber), working around the circumference until you reach the seeds in the centre, which should be discarded or composted.

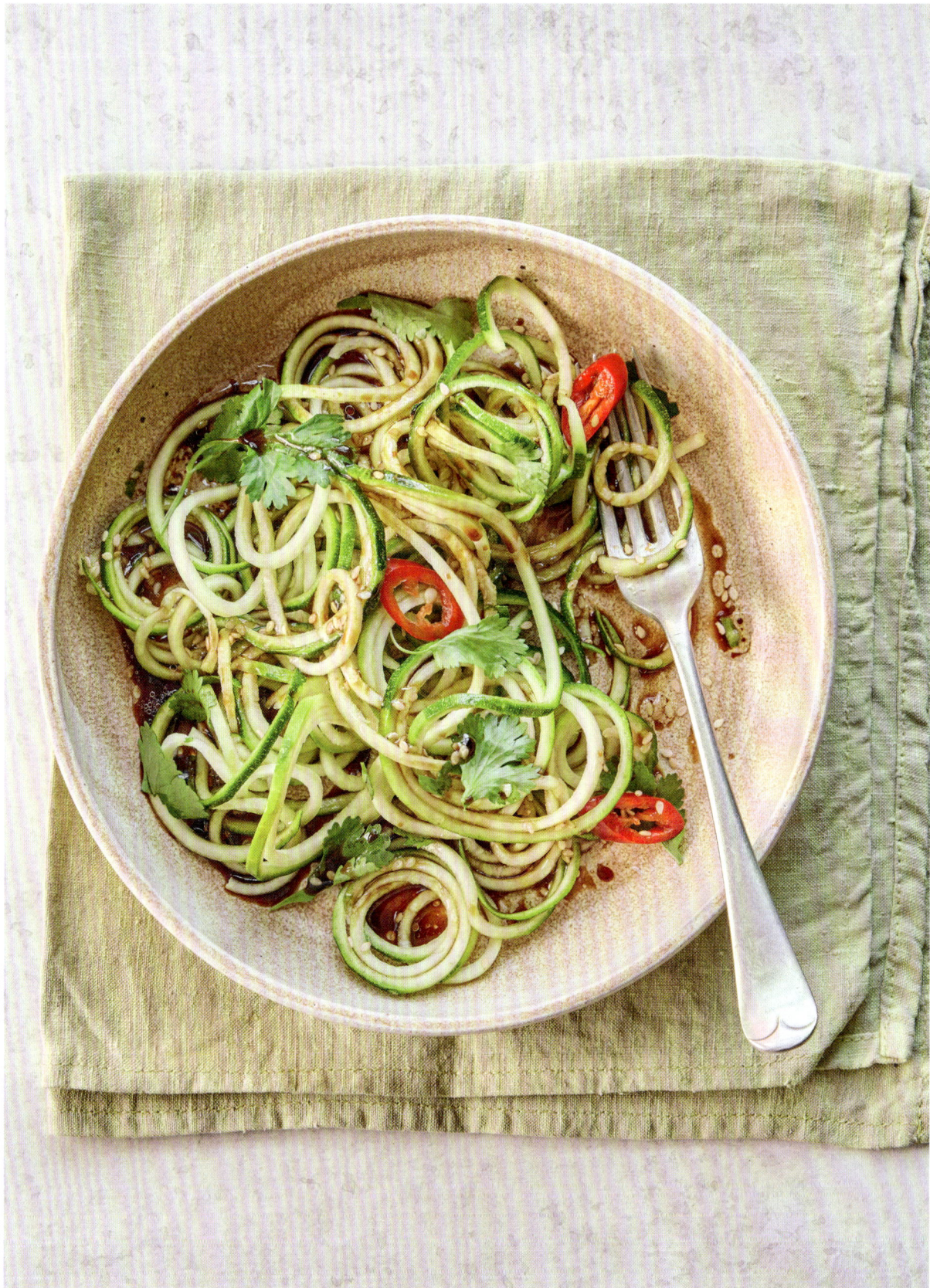

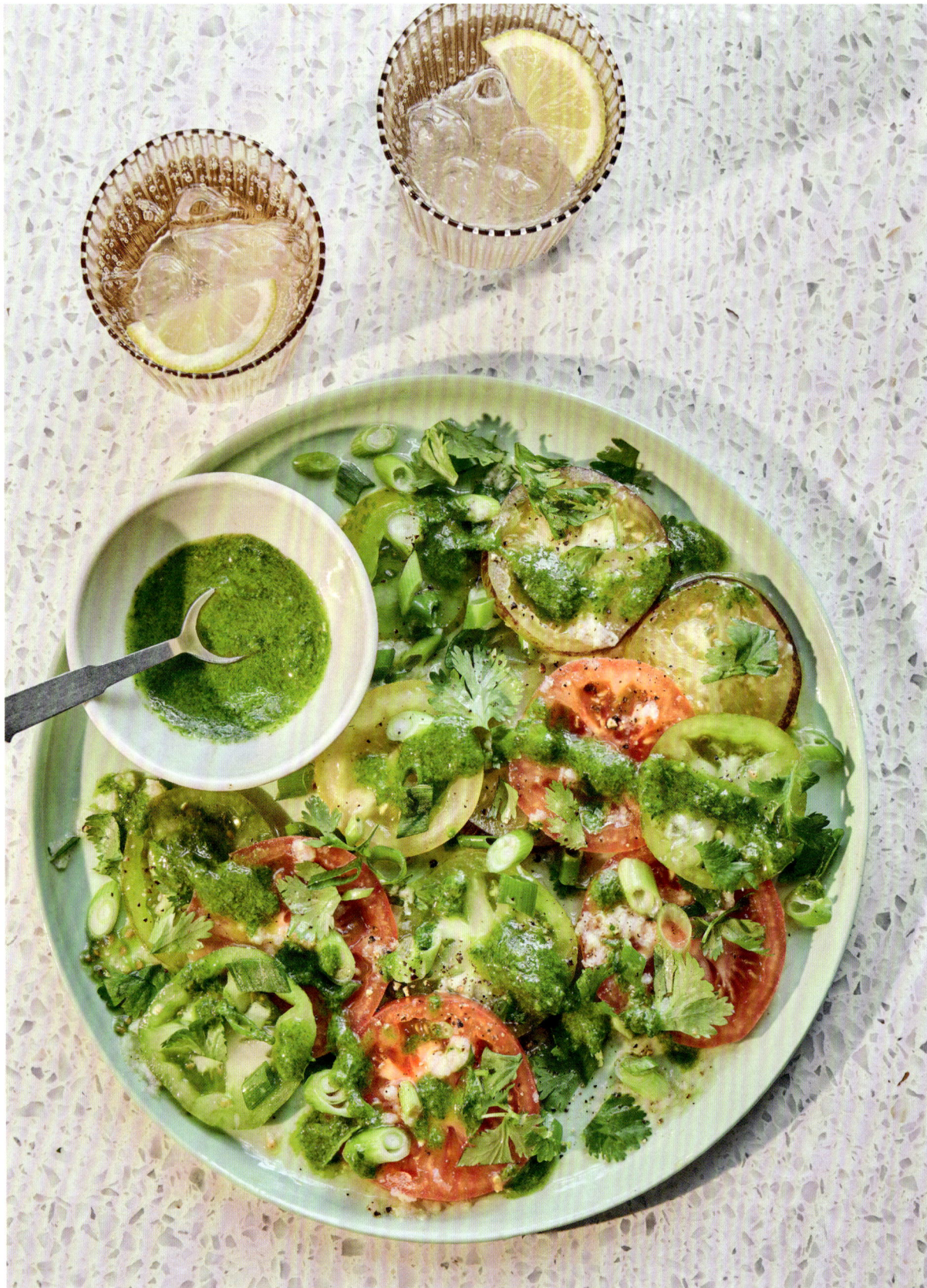

SUMMER TOMATO SALAD
WITH SALSA VERDE

SERVES
2

PREP TIME
10 MINS

170g (6oz) tomatoes, cut into slices or wedges (or halved, if using cherry tomatoes)

3 garlic cloves, crushed, or 2–3 teaspoons garlic purée, to taste

30g (1oz) shallot, red onion or spring onions, finely chopped

2 tablespoons chopped fresh coriander leaves

2 teaspoons olive oil

1 tablespoon lime juice

cracked black pepper

For the salsa verde

2 teaspoons olive oil

2 teaspoons apple cider vinegar

1 teaspoon capers, finely chopped

1 small garlic clove, crushed

2 tablespoons finely chopped flat leaf parsley leaves

2 tablespoons finely chopped basil leaves

2 tablespoons finely chopped mint leaves

sea salt flakes

A very quick, colourful and tangy plate combining flavour, texture and taste. Preparing the dish a few hours in advance of serving allows the garlic to infuse with the tomato, but if you're short on time, it isn't necessary. This is fantastic alongside grilled fish, or a juicy steak, once you are in Step 3. In Step 1, a portion is 2 teaspoons of salsa verde with half the tomato salad.

1 To make the salsa verde, whizz the oil, vinegar, capers, garlic and some salt in the small bowl of a food processor. Add the chopped herbs and blend until smooth. Alternatively, finely chop everything by hand and mix together to achieve a smooth consistency.

2 To make the salad, place the tomatoes, garlic and shallot or onion in a bowl and mix together to combine. Add all the other tomato salad ingredients.

3 If following Step 2 or Step 3, stir the salsa verde into the tomato salad. (For Step 1, follow the portioning advice in the recipe introduction.)

4 Serve with a generous twist of cracked black pepper.

PER SERVING	
NET CARBS	4.8G
FIBRE	2.4G
PROTEIN	1.8G
FAT	8.7G
KCAL	115

GREEK SALAD WITH DILL AND MINT

SERVES
3

PREP TIME
15 MINS

200g (7oz) cherry tomatoes, quartered

½ red onion, finely sliced

1 cucumber, quartered and finely sliced

50g (1¾oz) olives, pitted and halved

2 tablespoons capers

1 green pepper, deseeded and finely sliced

spray of olive oil

sea salt flakes

For the dressing

1 tablespoon olive oil

1 tablespoon lemon juice

2 teaspoons apple cider vinegar

1 tablespoon finely chopped dill

1 tablespoon finely chopped mint leaves

freshly ground black pepper

I have always loved Greek salads, they are so bright and colourful and contain just the right balance of flavour and crunch. The combination of herbs here really elevates the flavours of the fresh vegetables, while capers add a salty twist. This is the perfect plate to enjoy with your smoothies in Step 1, or as a side dish in Steps 2 or 3.

1 To make the salad, place the tomatoes, red onion and cucumber in a mixing bowl and season with salt and pepper.

2 Add the olives, capers and green pepper to the bowl. Spray with a little olive oil and lightly toss everything together.

3 To make the dressing, combine the olive oil, lemon juice, apple cider vinegar, chopped dill and mint and season with pepper in a small bowl, then whisk with a fork. Alternatively, place in a clean jam jar, put the lid on and shake vigorously.

4 Pour the dressing over the salad and toss everything together, then serve immediately.

PER SERVING	
NET CARBS	8.3G
FIBRE	4G
PROTEIN	3.4G
FAT	7.7G
KCAL	128

RECIPE TIP
You could serve this salad with Baked Lemon and Garlic Salmon Parcels or Marinated Chicken Kebabs (see pages 138 and 157). Alternatively, it would make a good light lunch with a can of oily fish such as sardines or mackerel, or some roasted chickpeas (see page 118) would be a nutritious and convenient option.

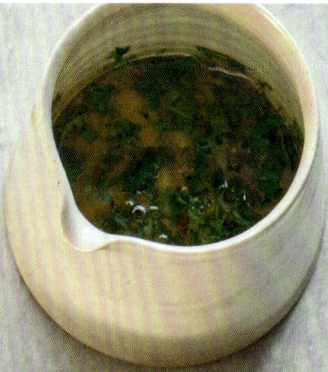

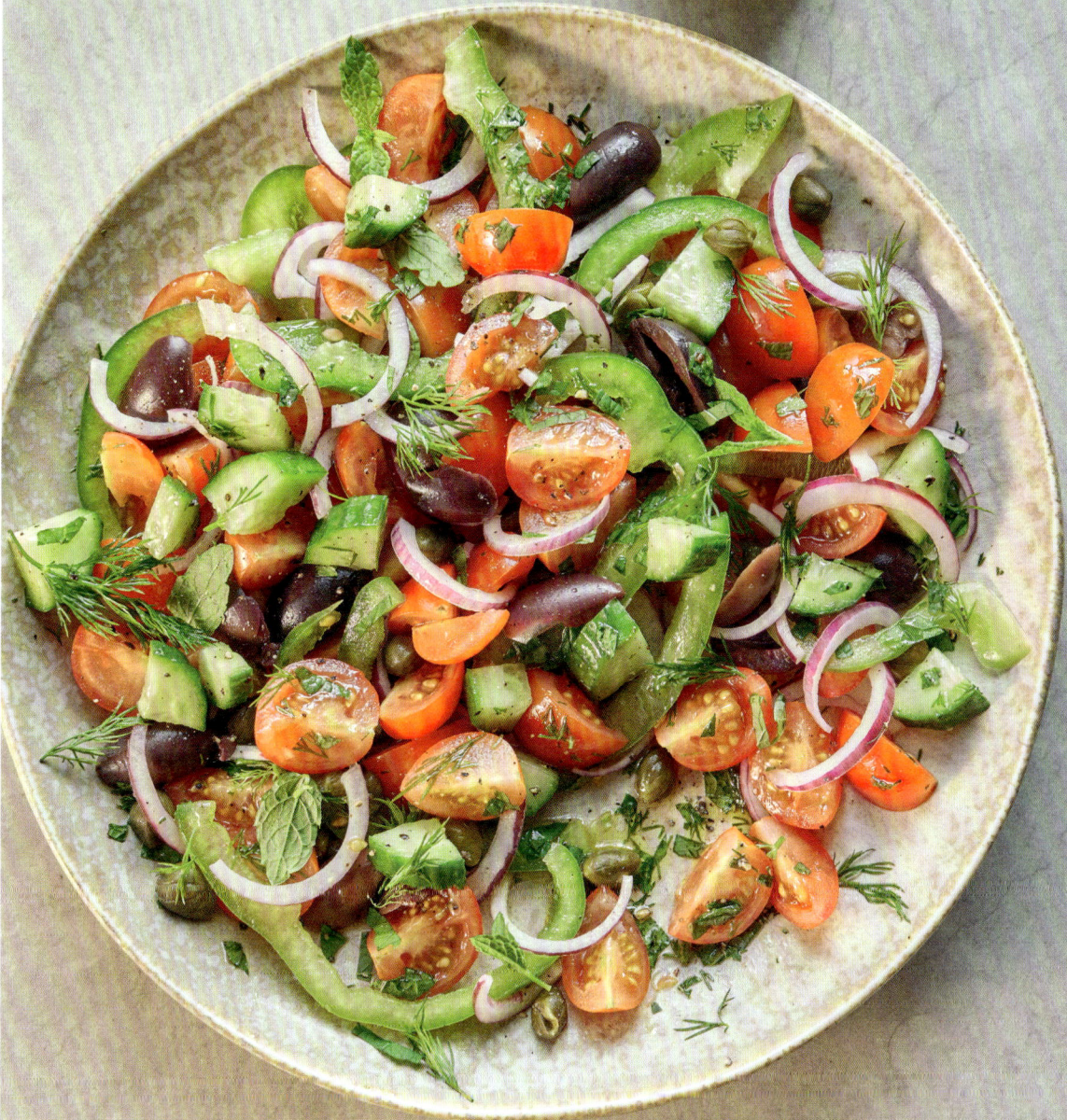

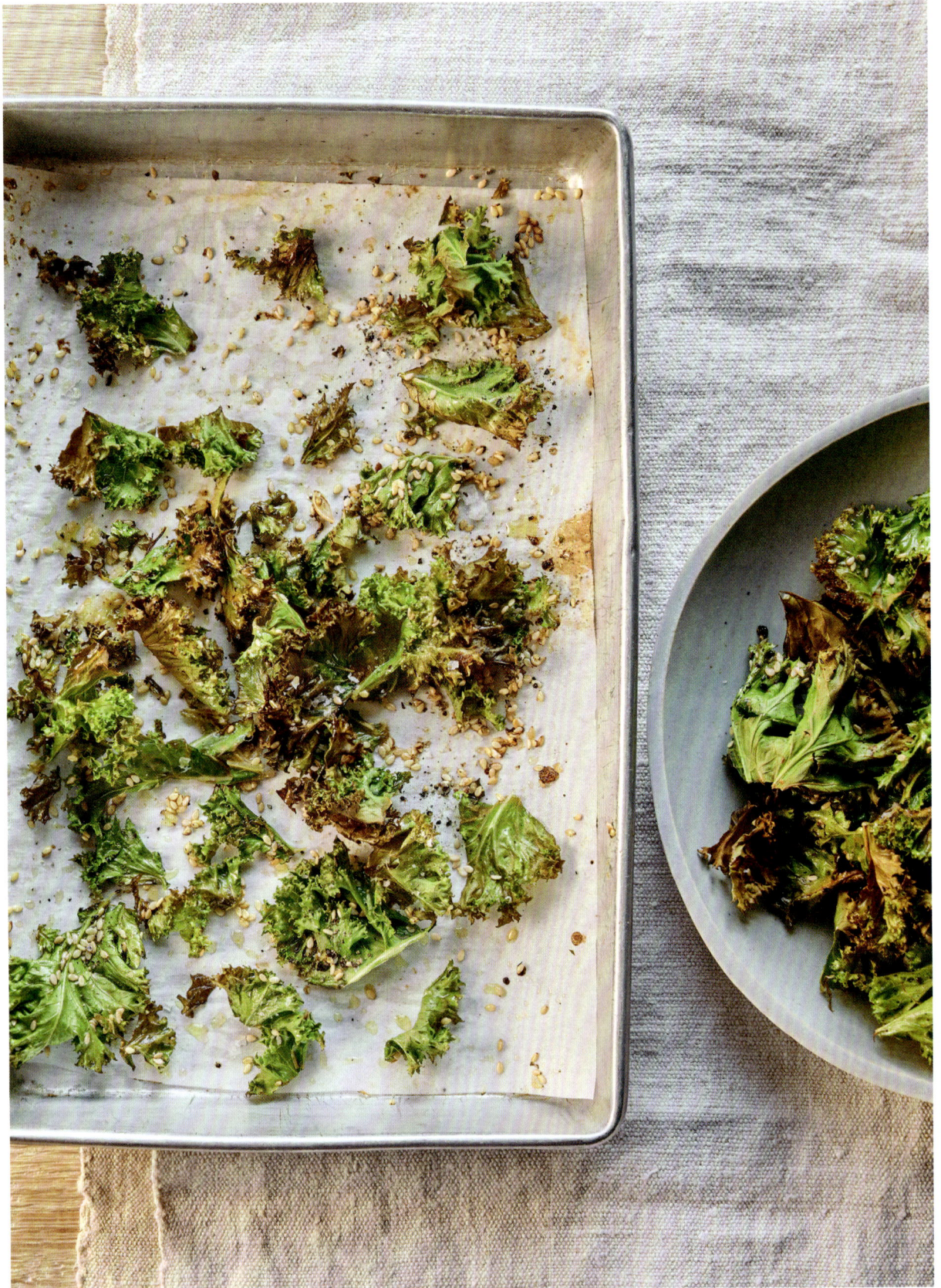

LEMON AND SESAME KALE CRISPS

SERVES
3

PREP TIME
5 MINS

COOK TIME
12 MINS

150g (5½oz) curly kale, coarse stalks removed

olive oil

juice of ½ lemon

2 teaspoons sesame seeds

1 teaspoon sea salt flakes

PER SERVING	
NET CARBS	0.8G
FIBRE	2.39G
PROTEIN	2.2G
FAT	5.1G
KCAL	64

A great way to enjoy something crunchy and delicious, while benefitting from a healthy dose of fibre. These are tangy and extremely satisfying. Keep them in an airtight container for up to 5 days.

1 Preheat the oven to 170°C (340°F), Gas Mark 3½. Have 2 baking sheets ready.

2 The kale must be completely dry, so dry it on a tea towel if it's wet from washing. Place it in a large bowl and add a small drizzle of olive oil and the lemon juice. With your hands, massage the oil and lemon juice into the leaves until they are completely coated.

3 Sprinkle in most of the sesame seeds and toss with the kale to ensure an even spread.

4 Place half the kale on each baking sheet and spread out evenly. If you can, try to create a small space between the leaves. Scatter the remaining sesame seeds on top and the salt all over.

5 Place in the oven for 10–12 minutes, until the edges are browning very slightly and the kale is a dark green. Be careful, as if they are left for too long the crisps will burn very quickly!

RECIPE TIP

All ovens vary, so please keep a close eye on your kale crisps, as the last thing you want is for them to burn. If you have an air fryer, you can halve the cooking time to 6 minutes at the same temperature.

CRUDITÉS

SERVES
4

PREP TIME
10 MINS

300g (10½oz) carrots

300g (10½oz) celery

200g (7oz) cucumber

200g (7oz) broccoli

50g (1¾oz) radishes

PER SERVING	
NET CARBS	9.2G
FIBRE	6.5G
PROTEIN	3.5G
FAT	1G
KCAL	73

Crudités are a fantastic snack, as they are low in both calories and carbs. They provide an excellent source of fibre and are bright, vibrant and crunchy. Enjoy a portion with 2 tablespoons of a homemade dip (see pages 68–71): the crunch alongside something smooth and tasty is a delicious way to enjoy crudités. Alternatively, 1 tablespoon of low-salt soy sauce works as a low-calorie dip, too.

1 Peel and cut your vegetables into finger-friendly pieces.

2 You can peel and cut the vegetables up to 1 day ahead of time and keep them in peak condition submerged in a bowl of cold water in the refrigerator.

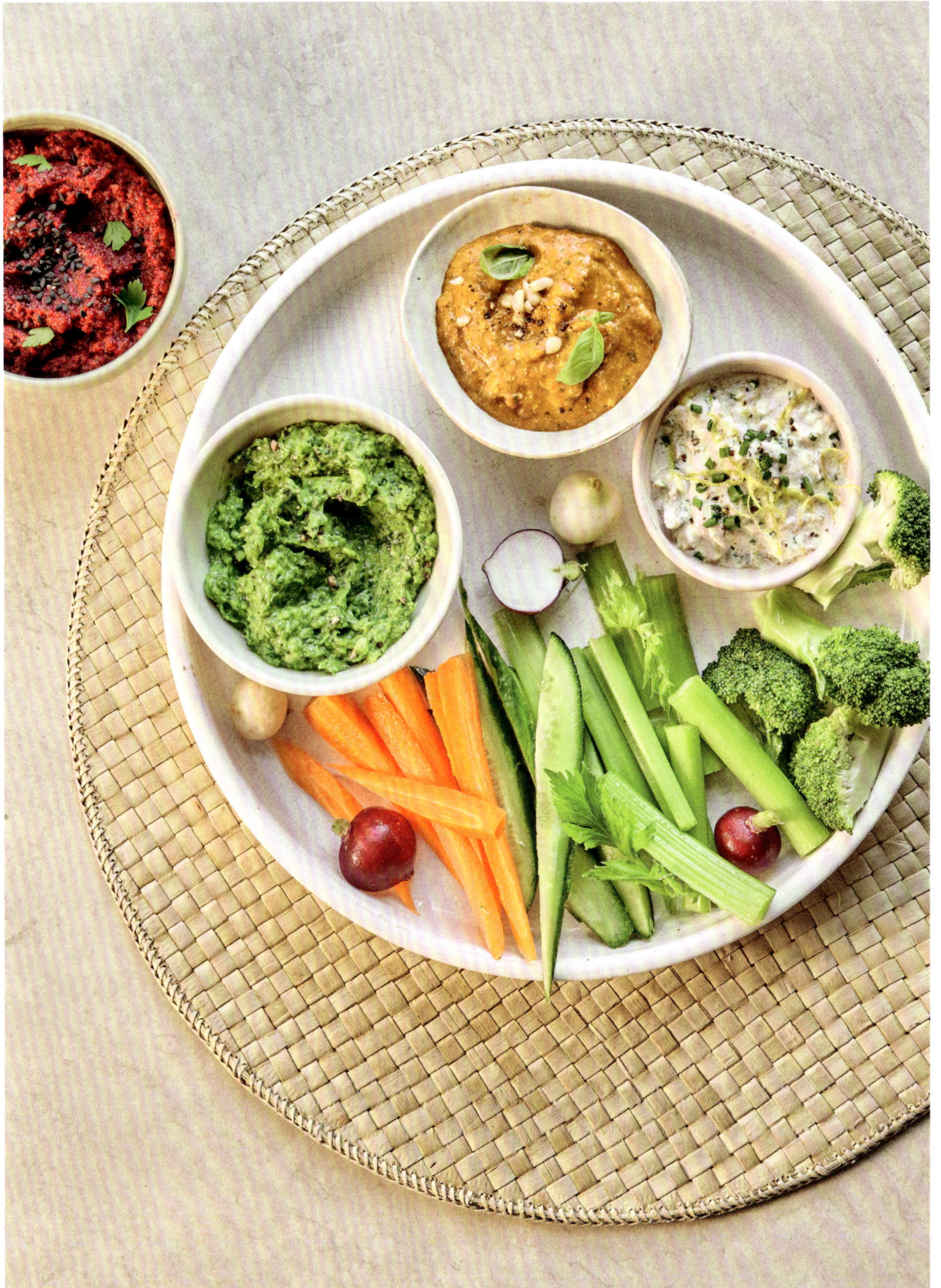

DIPS 4 WAYS
KALE, GARLIC AND AVOCADO CREAM

SERVES
4 (2 TABLESPOONS PER SERVING)

PREP TIME
5 MINS

2 handfuls of kale, coarse stalks removed

1 avocado, peeled and pitted

juice of ½ lime

1 garlic clove

sea salt flakes and cracked black pepper

Smooth and peppery, this is a really memorable dip that's full of flavour; a great way to enjoy kale.

1 Place the kale in a food processor and finely chop.

2 Add a splash of water, the avocado, lime juice, garlic, a pinch of salt and ½ teaspoon cracked black pepper. Blend on full speed until smooth and creamy.

3 If the dip is too thick, gradually add a little more water.

4 Place in an airtight container in the refrigerator for up to 3 days.

PER SERVING	
NET CARBS	0.9G
FIBRE	1.7G
PROTEIN	1.1G
FAT	6.3G
KCAL	69

LOW-STARCH VEGETABLE PLATES

MACKEREL AND CREAMY CHIVE DIP

SERVES
3

PREP TIME
5 MINS

1 90g (3¼oz) can of mackerel fillets in olive oil

1 teaspoon finely grated lemon zest, plus more to serve

1 tablespoon lemon juice

50g (1¾oz) soured cream

2 tablespoons chopped chives, plus more to serve

sea salt flakes and freshly ground black pepper

PER SERVING	
NET CARBS	0.6G
FIBRE	0G
PROTEIN	6.9G
FAT	8.8G
KCAL	109

Oily fish is a great source of lean protein and is full of minerals such as iron, zinc, selenium and iodine, plus vitamins A and D. The essential omega 3 fatty acids it contains have been shown to have a positive impact on heart health, cognitive function and joint mobility, and they also play a key role in hormone production and defending against some chronic diseases. Here, the salty mackerel and the oniony chives combine to make a really stunning dip, a perfect topping for my Multiseed Crackers (see page 178), as well as for a dip for crudités (see page 66).

1 Place the mackerel, its oil, the lemon zest and juice in a bowl and carefully mix together, breaking up the mackerel into smaller pieces.

2 Add the soured cream, chives, 1 teaspoon sea salt flakes and some black pepper and stir to combine until creamy.

3 Place in a small serving bowl. Scatter with chives, lemon zest and a twist of black pepper. Keep refrigerated in a sealed container and consume within 2 days.

RECIPE TIP

Canned fish is widely available and good value. If you prefer to use a different oily fish in this recipe, you could opt for sardines or salmon. Anchovies can work too, but they are very salty.

LOW-STARCH VEGETABLE PLATES

ROASTED RED PEPPER PESTO

SERVES
4 (2 TABLESPOONS PER SERVING)

PREP TIME
10 MINS

COOK TIME
20 MINS

2 red peppers, halved and deseeded

2–3 tablespoons extra virgin olive oil

40g (1½oz) pine nuts, or other nuts of your choice

1 large handful of basil leaves

juice of ½ lemon

sea salt flakes and freshly ground black pepper

PER SERVING	
NET CARBS	4.1G
FIBRE	2.2G
PROTEIN	2.4G
FAT	16G
KCAL	180

An incredibly flavourful recipe that requires a little planning and prep, but the end result is so worth it. Not only is this a wonderful dip, it also makes a fantastic sauce for courgette 'noodles' (see page 58): a perfect twist on the classic carb-and-calorie-dense pesto pasta.

1 Preheat the oven to 180°C (350°F), Gas Mark 4. Line a baking sheet with nonstick baking paper.

2 Spray or rub the peppers with the oil, place on the prepared baking sheet and bake for about 20 minutes until soft and the skins have browned.

3 Transfer the peppers to a blender and add all the other ingredients with ½ teaspoon each of salt and pepper. Blitz for about 1 minute until fully combined and paste-like in texture. You might have to scrape down the sides of the bowl a couple of times during the process.

4 Serve straight away, or keep in an airtight container in the refrigerator for up to 3 days.

ROASTED BEETROOT HUMMUS

SERVES
3

PREP TIME
10 MINS

COOK TIME
40 MINS

4 beetroot

1 tablespoon olive oil, plus more to
   serve

1 garlic clove, finely chopped or grated

1 tablespoon apple cider vinegar

30g (1oz) tahini

juice of 1 small lemon

½ teaspoon ground cumin

100g (3½oz) canned chickpeas in
   water, drained

sea salt flakes

To serve (optional)

black sesame seeds

chopped parsley, fresh coriander
   or mint leaves

PER SERVING	
NET CARBS	10.9G
FIBRE	3.9G
PROTEIN	5G
FAT	11G
KCAL	165

A nutritionally dense dip which is incredibly creamy and looks as beautiful as it tastes; people always ask for the recipe when I serve this. It has such a depth of flavour and is perfect with crudités or Multiseed Crackers (see page 178). (Plus my young daughters adore it because it's Barbie-pink!) You should get into the habit of roasting beetroot regularly, then keep them in the refrigerator, ready to use for this recipe, for a soup (see page 54), or to add to a salad. When roasted, they keep for up to 5 days.

1 Preheat the oven to 180°C (350°F), Gas Mark 4.

2 Place the beetroot on a sheet of foil. Spray or rub with the olive oil and loosely wrap in the foil to make a parcel with space inside for the heat to circulate. Roast for 40 minutes or until a knife easily passes through the beetroot. When cool enough to handle, rub off the skins.

3 Put the beetroot and garlic into a food processor and blend until it has a crumbly consistency.

4 Add all the remaining ingredients with 1½ teaspoons of salt and continue to blend until creamy, using a spatula to scrape down the sides and pulse-blending until combined. If it seems too dry, add 1 tablespoon of water at a time until the desired consistency is reached. Taste and adjust the seasoning.

5 Transfer to a small serving dish and decorate with a drizzle of olive oil, a few black sesame seeds and chopped herbs, if you like. Keep refrigerated in a sealed container and consume within 4 days.

LOW-STARCH VEGETABLE PLATES

Moving on to
STEP

TWO

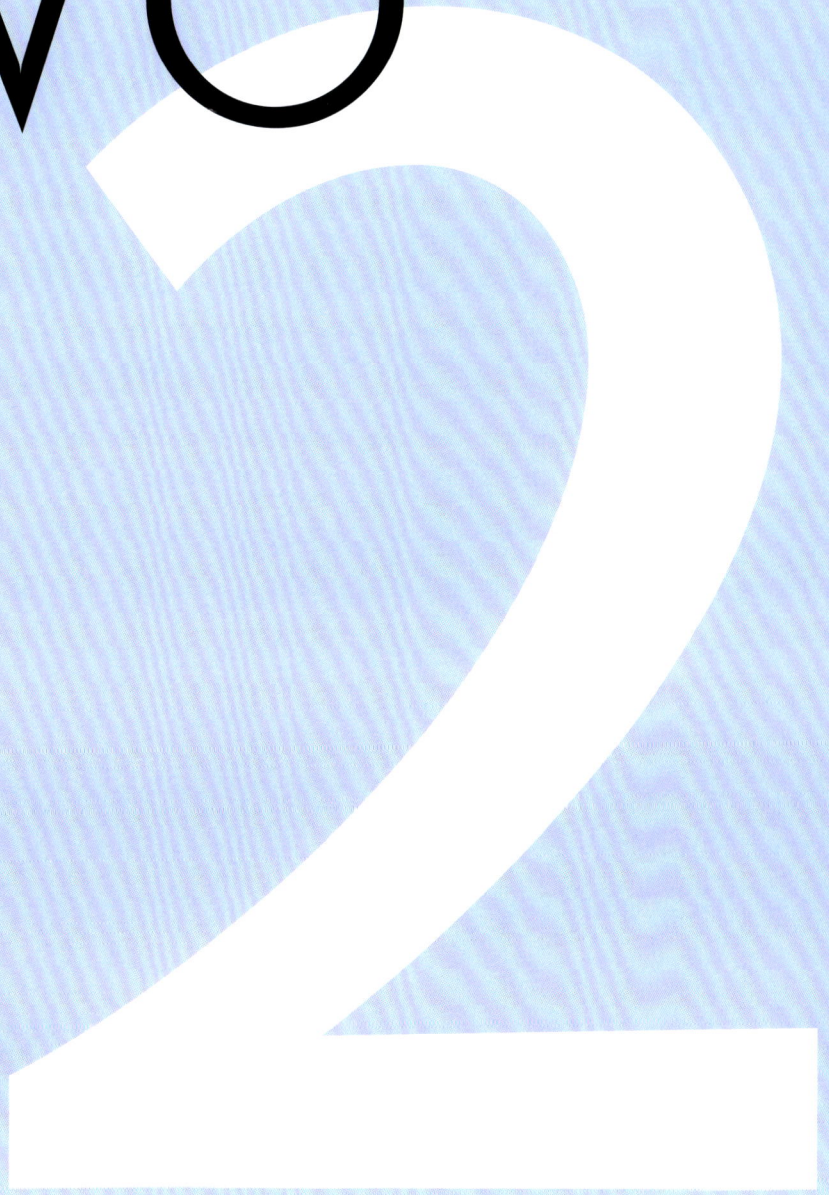

During Step 2, you will be gradually replacing the shakes and soups with solid foods. This will return you to a sustainable pattern of eating over a period of 3–6 weeks, during which time your weight should remain largely steady. This is done by introducing meals to replace shakes and soups, one meal at a time. The meals should still be low in carbohydrates and you should avoid sweet foods. Starchy foods such as potato, rice, pasta and bread should be consumed sparingly.

How long Step 2 takes is entirely down to you as an individual. This step should not be rushed, as it will set the scene for a lifelong pattern of eating. It could take you two weeks, it could take you six weeks or longer, so just relax into it. Remember to take things slowly: you have come this far and hopefully are starting to reap the rewards of type 2 diabetes remission and / or weight loss.

It can be challenging to start deciding what solid food to eat. To keep things as simple as possible, I recommend you begin with the low-starch vegetable plates from Step 1 (see pages 56–71) or your favourite salad, and simply add a portion of protein (see opposite). For example, you could have Greek Salad with Dill and Mint (see page 62) with 2 medium boiled eggs or a can of sardines, or Tangy Courgette 'Noodles' with Coriander, Chilli, Soy and Sesame (see page 58) with 75g (2½oz) cooked king prawns or 100g (3½oz) cooked tempeh.

HOW MUCH IS A PORTION OF PROTEIN?

- 2 medium eggs: 130 kcal

- 100g (3½oz) chicken breast: 165 kcal

- 75g (2½oz) cooked king prawns: 65 kcal

- 75g (2½oz) cottage cheese: 83 kcal

- 1 can (145g / 5oz) tuna in water, drained: 115 kcal

- 1 can (125g / 4½oz) mackerel in water, drained: 200 kcal

- 1 can (120g / 4¼oz) sardines in water, drained: 175 kcal

- 100g (3½oz) tempeh: 195 kcal

- 100g (3½oz) lentils, boiled and drained: 142 kcal

- 100g (3½oz) edamame beans: 105 kcal

- 100g (3½oz) firm tofu: 120 kcal

- 150g (5½oz) chickpeas: 230 kcal

During Step 2, you can replace a smoothie, shake or soup with a meal for either lunch (400 kcal) or dinner (400–500 kcal). Continue following this regime until you have reached your target weight.

When you are feeling kitchen- and cooking-confident, look to include recipes from other sections of this book, such as Chickpea Dal or Thai Turkey Burgers (see pages 129 and 150). These recipes serve three or four people, so you can eat one portion, freeze a couple of others and save the last for the next day.

Focus on making healthy food choices, cooking from scratch, and always ensuring you have prepped ahead and have a nutritious meal to hand, even if it has been a hectic day.

Continue to follow the steps in the How to use this book section (see page 26) and **BE PROUD OF YOURSELF.**

How to build a salad

In order to truly enjoy a salad and feel satisfied, it's a good idea to follow a few simple rules. Your salad should look appetizing, have texture and crunch, taste good and – most importantly – you should want to make it and eat it again!

Salads can be eaten at any time of day and, though they're best when freshly prepared, they can be popped into a reusable jar or airtight container and enjoyed on the go. Preparing a salad the night before you need it means that you will be far less likely to succumb to ultra-processed convenience food – undoubtedly worse both for your health and your bank balance – when lunchtime rolls around.

When it comes to salads, they're often thought of as a healthy option to help you lose weight. However, while salads can be incredibly healthy and a fantastic way to boost your nutrient intake, this is not always the case. If you find yourself adding dressings, simple carbohydrates such as rice or pasta, sauces or fried toppings, they can very quickly turn from a quick, nutritious plate into a calorie-packed meal that may contribute to weight gain. However, eating only a few salad leaves or low-starch veggies (lettuce and tomato, I'm looking at you!) may leave you feeling hungry again very quickly.

So here's how to build a better salad that will allow you to reap the health benefits. The beauty of salads is that they're so adaptable to using up a variety of ingredients usually already in the refrigerator. You can create a salad out of almost anything: just be mindful of the quantity and quality of the food.

1. First, your base
A good rule of thumb is to start with a couple of large handfuls of washed leafy greens, such as rocket, chicory, Swiss chard, watercress, spinach or Romaine lettuce. Packs of pre-washed salad leaves and bistro salad mixes are brilliant, too: not only are they convenient but full of nutrients and fibre.

2. Add a portion of protein
The downfall of many salads is that they're lacking in protein, which can often be why they don't keep you feeling full for very long. Not only does protein help to curb cravings, but it is very important for growth, repair and the maintenance of muscle mass. Here are some high-protein options you could add:

1 large egg: 78 kcal

100g (3½oz) chicken breast: 165 kcal

75g (2¾oz) cooked king prawns: 65 kcal

75g (2¾oz) cottage cheese: 83 kcal

160g (5¾oz) can of tuna in water, drained: 115 kcal

100g (3½oz) tempeh: 195 kcal

100g (3½oz) lentils, boiled: 142 kcal

100g (3½oz) edamame beans: 105 kcal

100g (3½oz) firm tofu: 120 kcal

3. A portion of healthy fats
Fats will help keep you fuller for longer and also add flavour to your salads. You can find plenty of healthy fats in extra virgin olive oil, avocados, nuts and seeds, all fantastic additions to a salad.

It is important to be mindful of portion sizes when it comes to adding fats, as they are higher in calories:

½ avocado (70g / 2½oz): 145 kcal

10g (¼oz) mixed nuts: 65 kcal

10g (¼oz) mixed seeds: 60 kcal

20g (¾oz) feta cheese: 50 kcal

1 tablespoon olive oil: 120 kcal

4. A little texture
Crunchy veg such as carrots, sugar snap peas, gherkins or radishes add texture and can really satisfy cravings. Fermented foods such as sauerkraut – with its wonderful crunch – are a delicious addition, too.

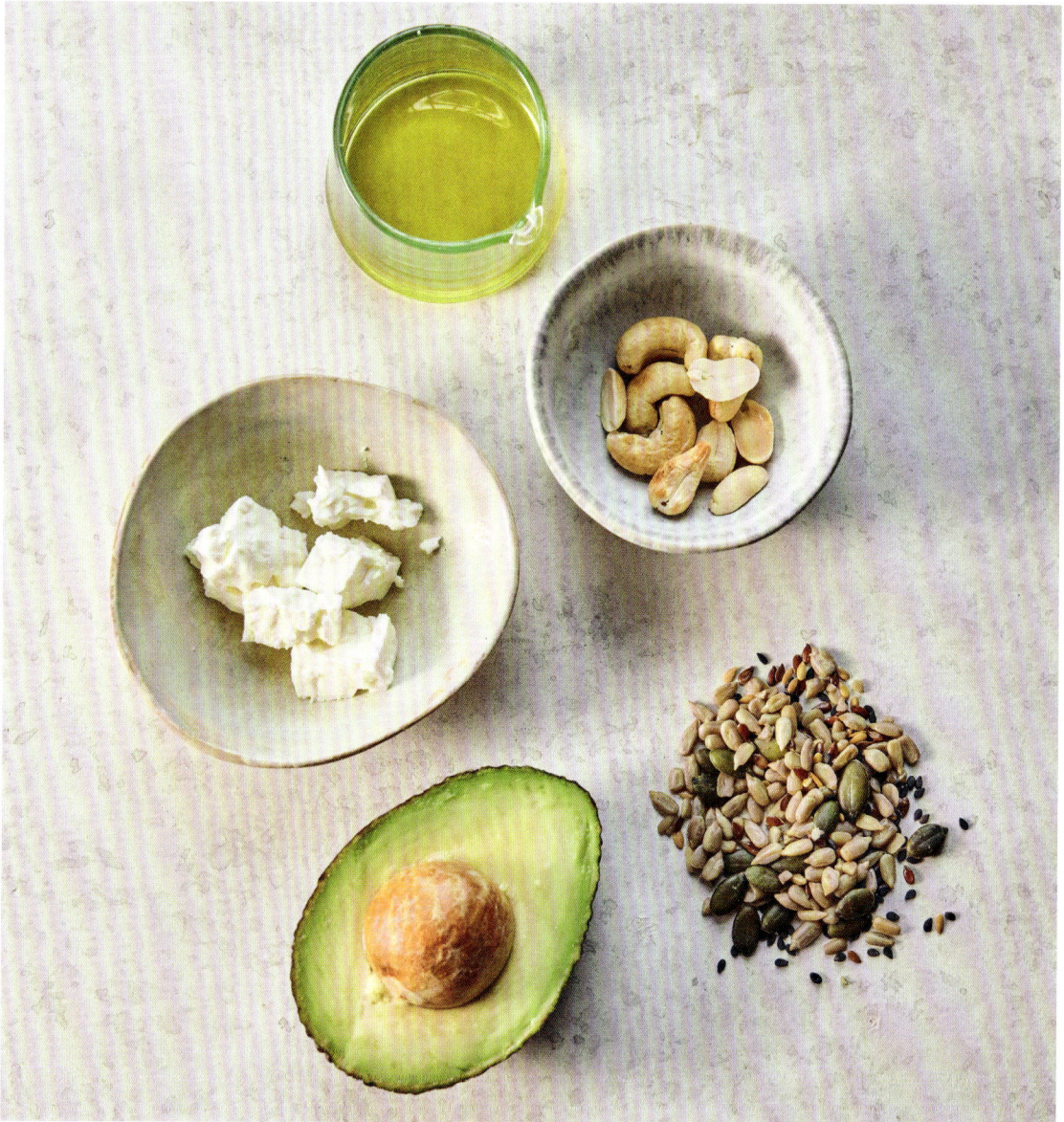

5. A pop of colour

The more colours you have on your plate, the more nutrients there will be in the food.

Eating seasonably available foods (as far as possible) helps to keep food costs down, or you might even be able to grow vegetables yourself to add to your plate. Colourful peppers or tomatoes add plenty of vitamins and minerals to your salad. Low-starch vegetables can be eaten freely on the 1-2-3 plan without the need to count their calories, so feel free to use plenty, which will also help you to feel satiated.

RECIPE TIP

Use a spray bottle to add olive oil to your salad: you will still reap the benefits, but reduce the calories significantly. (See page 17 for more on spray bottles and olive oil.)

6. Low-starch vegetables

These are a good source of dietary fibre, which aids digestion, especially when you are on a low-calorie diet. You can create many exciting dishes with low-starch vegetables (see pages 56–71).

Learn more about low-starch vegetables, on pages 82–5.

Artichoke hearts, without oil	Courgettes	Parsley
Asparagus	Cucumbers	Pea shoots
Aubergines	Fennel	Peppers
Baby corn	Frozen vegetable mixes	Pickles (unsweetened)
Bamboo shoots	Garlic	Pumpkins
Basil	Ginger	Radishes
Beetroot greens	Green beans	Romaine lettuce
Beetroot	Green leaf lettuce	Rosemary
Bok choi	Hearts of palm	Sauerkraut
Broccoli	Iceberg lettuce	Shallots
Brussels sprouts	Jalapeño peppers	Spinach
Butternut squash	Kale	Spring onions
Cabbage	Leeks	Sugar snap peas
Carrots	Lettuce	Summer squash
Cauliflower	Mint	Swiss chard
Celeriac	Mixed salad leaves	Tarragon
Celery	Mushrooms	Thyme
Chillies	Mustard greens	Tomatoes
Chives	Nori (dried seaweed)	Turnips
Collard greens	Onions	Watercress
Coriander	Oregano	

7. Lastly, some flavour

Try not to drench your salad in dressing, or to use shop-bought dressings laden with sugar, additives and preservatives. Dressings don't have to be fancy – in fact, they are absolutely delicious created from just a few ingredients, which you'll probably already have in your cupboards. You can keep it simple with a drizzle of extra virgin olive oil, apple cider vinegar, wholegrain mustard or a squeeze of lemon juice, or try the Simple Basil Vinaigrette recipe, opposite. Remember, also, to add fresh herbs. Coriander – if you like it – can really lift a salad, adding freshness and zing.

HOW TO BUILD A SALAD

SIMPLE BASIL VINAIGRETTE

MAKES
ABOUT 10 TABLESPOONS

PREP TIME
5 MINS

8 tablespoons olive oil

2 handfuls of basil leaves, chopped

1 garlic clove, crushed and finely
chopped

finely grated zest and juice of
½ lemon, plus more to taste

sea salt and freshly ground black
pepper

PER TABLESPOON	
NET CARBS	0.3G
FIBRE	TRACE
PROTEIN	0G
FAT	10G
KCAL	93

Make this, pop it in a spray bottle and use it throughout the week.
It works out at about 5 kcal per spray.

1 Place all the ingredients in a bowl with ½ teaspoon salt and a grind of
pepper and whisk until fully combined. Taste and adjust the flavours
with more lemon juice or salt if you like.

2 Pour into a spray bottle and keep in the refrigerator for whenever
required. The longer you leave it, the more the flavours will infuse, but
always give the bottle a little shake before use.

Salad in a jar 3 ways

To create salad jars, add the ingredients to your jar or airtight container in the following order:

1 DRESSING INGREDIENTS / LIQUID

2 PROTEIN

3 CRUNCHY, LOW-STARCH VEG (SEE PAGE 78)

4 EXTRA CRUNCH

5 LEAVES

This way, the leaves stay crisp and fresh until the jar is upended on to a serving plate, and the dressing drizzles over everything at the end.

HOW TO BUILD A SALAD

VEGETARIAN

3 teaspoons Roasted Beetroot Hummus (see page 71)

100g (3½oz) edamame beans

2 teaspoons feta cheese

50g (1¾oz) roasted butternut squash

chopped cucumber, green pepper and pea shoots

toasted seeds

2 handfuls of mixed salad leaves

Layer each ingredient in you large jar or airtight container, then seal with a lid and refrigerate until ready to turn out and eat.

FISH

For the dressing

1 teaspoon olive oil

handful of finely chopped coriander leaves

1 teaspoon apple cider vinegar

1 teaspoon lime juice

1 teaspoon natural yogurt

For the salad

100g (3½oz) cooked salmon or cooked king prawns

spiralized courgette, chopped cucumber and finely sliced red onion

2 teaspoons cashew nuts

2 handfuls of spinach leaves

Mix all the dressing ingredients together in the base of your jar or airtight container. Add the salmon, courgette, nuts and spinach in layers, then seal with a lid and refrigerate until ready to turn out and eat.

MEAT

For the dressing

1 teaspoon peanut butter

1 teaspoon apple cider vinegar

1 teaspoon low-salt soy sauce

For the salad

100g (3½oz) cooked chicken breast, sliced

raw shredded cabbage, grated carrot and sliced spring onion

2 teaspoons unsalted peanuts

2 handfuls of rocket

Mix all the dressing ingredients together in the base of your jar or airtight container. Add the chicken, cabbage, peanuts and rocket in layers, then seal with a lid and refrigerate until ready to turn out and eat.

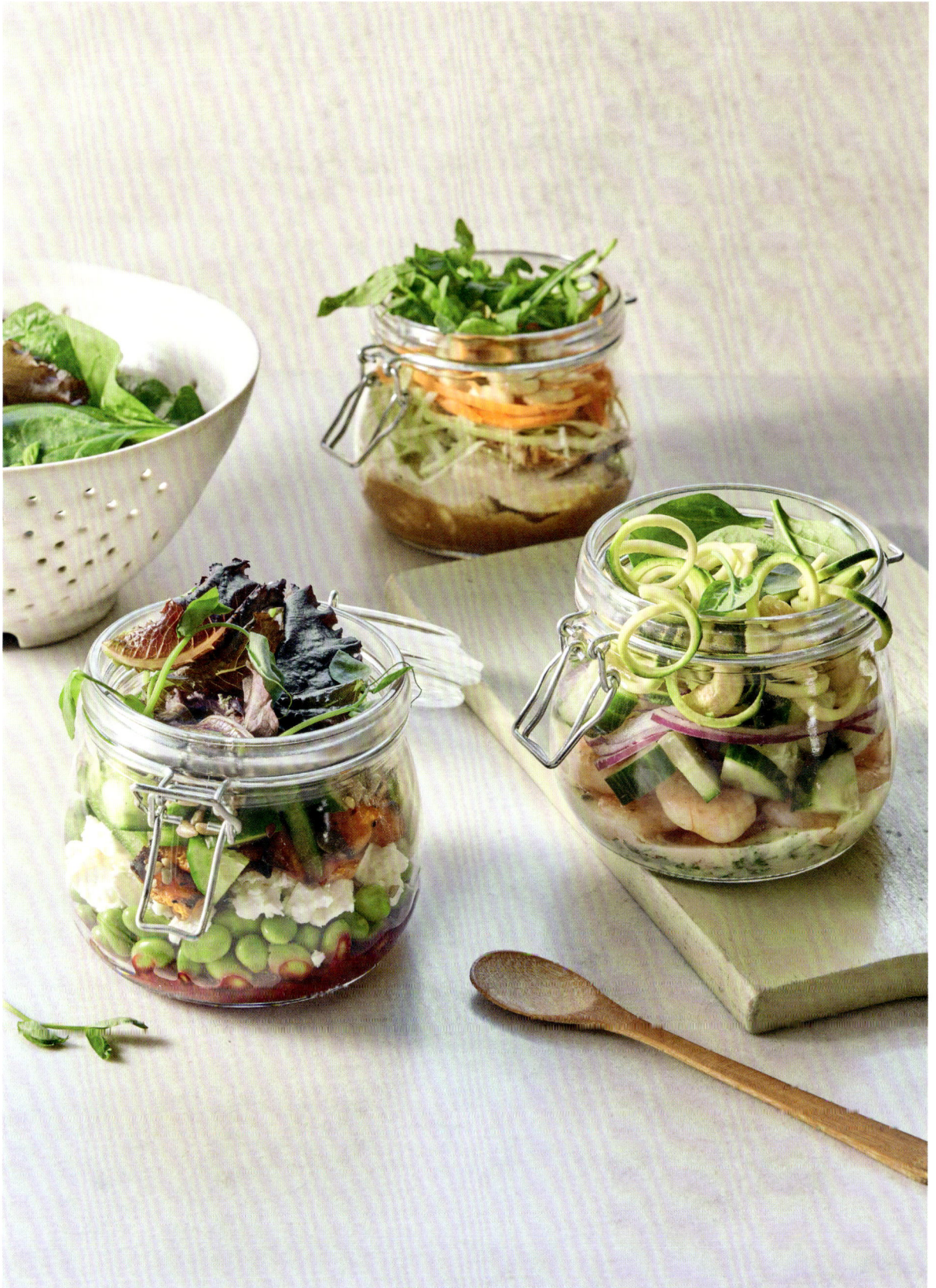

Love your low-starch vegetables

Low-starch vegetables (see page 78) are an excellent option, particularly because they are lower in carbs too, making them an excellent food choice for keeping blood sugars balanced and for those who are looking to consume fewer calories. By shifting the focus to flavouring, cooking and enhancing low-starch veg, this can be a game-changer for people managing diabetes or watching their calorie intake. Incorporating more low-starch veg into your diet can be a simple, effective way to support blood sugar management, nutrient intake and help with weight control.

Low-starch vegetables are incredibly beneficial for several reasons:

LOW IN CALORIES

This means you can eat larger portions to create a feeling of fullness, while keeping overall calorie intake in check.

HIGH IN FIBRE

Fibre adds bulk to your meals and promotes feelings of fullness. Soluble fibre also slows down digestion, helping to stabilize blood sugar levels (for those without insulin-dependent diabetes) and reduce cravings.

NUTRIENT DENSE

Low-starch vegetables are packed with essential vitamins, minerals and antioxidants, which are important for overall health and wellbeing. By incorporating a variety of colourful vegetables into your diet, you can ensure you are eating a wide range of nutrients.

LOW IN CARBS

Low-starch vegetables such as leafy greens, peppers, cabbage, cucumbers, broccoli and cauliflower are low in carbohydrates, meaning they have minimal impact on blood sugar levels. This makes them ideal for people with type 2 diabetes, as they prevent spikes in glucose.

HIGH WATER CONTENT

Not only will they contribute to hydration, they will help keep you feeling full and satisfied.

Ways to add flavour without the calories

Experiment and have fun with the food you are creating. You know what you like and what your tastes are, but be open-minded and try new things. You will find many of the foods below in your supermarket. Try investigating the international foods section, especially the pickled vegetables and delicious fermented foods.

Season with sea salt flakes, cracked black pepper, curry powder, chilli flakes, ground cumin or paprika.

Dry-fry cumin seeds, rosemary sprigs or nigella seeds to add to low-starch veg.

Very finely chopped garlic or sliced onions – including spring onion and chives – can add savoury flavour.

The finely grated zest and juice of lemon, lime or orange add a tangy flavour boost without too many calories.

Splash with low-salt soy sauce.

Freshly chopped herbs such as basil, mint, coriander, chives or dill can add a burst of fresh flavour.

Vinegar: pure balsamic vinegar, apple cider vinegar or red wine vinegar add acidity and flavour without many calories.

Pickled chillies, cucumber and cauliflower add crunch and flavour.

Fermented foods such as sauerkraut and kimchi contain fibre but are very low in calories, so they're great for adding to a dish on the side.

Miso is a low-calorie Japanese paste produced by fermenting soy beans. It's lovely as a low-calorie soup in a large cup or small bowl with some boiling water and sliced spring onions.

Dollop on some wholegrain mustard.

Ways to cook low-starch vegetables

Any of these cooking methods will work well for Steps 1, 2 and 3.

LOW-STARCH VEGETABLES

QUICK WOK STIR-FRY

Slice vegetables thinly or coarsely grate them to create a fantastic quick stir-fry, using a small amount of sesame oil or coconut oil to cook them. Stir-frying maintains the bright colours and crunchy texture. Serve with a portion of protein.

VEGETABLE 'NOODLES'

Use a spiralizer to make noodle alternatives; this works best with courgettes. (See page 58 for method.)

CRUDITÉS

Before eating any raw vegetables, make sure you wash them, even if you are going to peel them. Crudites are fresh, colourful raw vegetables, which are sliced and cut into easy finger food or eaten whole if they're small, such as radishes. They are ideal for dipping into sauces or homemade dips (see pages 68–71). Many vegetables can be enjoyed raw, but some are even better when they are lightly blanched, such as asparagus and green beans, a process which makes them more palatable and easier to digest. Just drop them into boiling water for 1–2 minutes, then drain and refresh in a bowl of cold water to stop the cooking.

ROASTING

Peel and chop all vegetables for roasting and bear in mind that some take longer to roast than others. Keeping a tub of roasted vegetables to hand in the refrigerator is a great way to quickly add flavour and fibre to your plate. Season with sea salt flakes and black pepper and enhance the flavours with garlic and other spices or herbs.

FRIES AND WEDGES

Low-starch veg can be used as a great substitute for conventional potato chips (see pages 114, 124 and 169) which are perfect for the whole family to enjoy. These are best served as a side dish alongside protein dishes such as Crispy Fish Goujons or Thai Turkey Burgers (see pages 141 and 150), to create a twist on the classic fish or chicken and chips.

VEGETABLE 'RICE'

Place cauliflower, broccoli, Brussels sprouts or cabbage in a food processor and pulse-blend to a rice-like consistency. You can elevate the flavour by adding garlic, ginger, sea salt flakes, herbs and spices. Cauliflower 'rice' is a good alternative to rice as it has a low calorie count and is incredibly low in carbs too. Once you've pulse-blended it, divide into 100g (3½oz) portions, place in freezer bags and freeze for up to 3 months. This will make life much easier, especially when you are hungry and need a quick accompaniment to a meal. No need to defrost first: heat a frying pan over a medium-low heat and add the frozen cauliflower 'rice' along with 1 teaspoon coconut oil, sea salt flakes and some ground cumin, and cook for 5 minutes – this is a delicious combination. Alternatively, add the 'rice' from frozen directly into stews, casseroles or soups and heat through.

Welcome to your 'new normal'

STEP

THREE

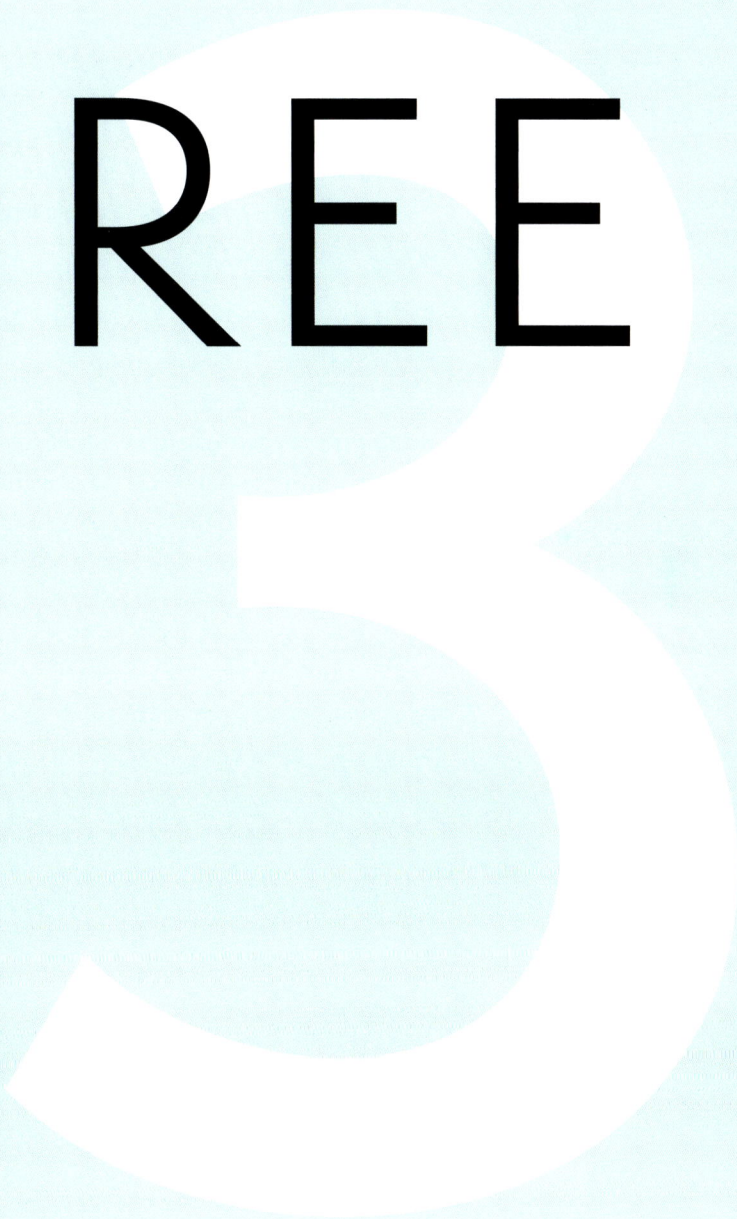

In this chapter, I've created a variety of recipes to inspire and entice you, and to help keep your blood sugars balanced. The recipes have been developed and finessed over the past decade, trialled during cookery classes, demonstrations and wellness retreats, as well as tested on family and friends, so I know they work brilliantly well. They use readily available ingredients that you should have no trouble sourcing in your local supermarkets or health food shops.

These are recipes to share with the people you love and, by using them, you will be able to maintain your weight loss, keep your diabetes in remission, or if you live with type 1 diabetes like me, help with blood sugar management while continuing to love food.

This is a lifestyle now. It is not a diet, it is not about counting calories and it does not restrict you from any food group. It is not about restriction, it is about control: blood sugar control and portion control. It is about maintaining your life without type 2 diabetes, or about having greater control of your type 1 diabetes. The overall goal is to avoid a long-term increase in weight. Use your weight measurements as a prompt to adjust the total amount you habitually eat.

Health is a reflection of how your body feels, of how you feel, both mentally and physically. Gone are the days of yearning to be skinny and jumping from one diet bandwagon to the next. Learn to just say 'no' to any kind offer of cake, biscuits or second helpings, because setting new habits is so important. Now you are focused on the future, on feeling well, satiated and in control. You can enjoy the delights of eating delicious food and sharing it with those you love.

'NEW NORMAL' TOP TIPS

- Cook from scratch, using whole, real food ingredients.

- Be active, whether by walking, gardening or higher-intensity exercises. Whatever you choose, do it because you enjoy it and reap the rewards.

- Stay hydrated: drink water.

- Prioritize sleep and minimize stress, where possible.

- Keep your carb intake down.

- Research intermittent fasting or time-restricted eating, and consider whether they will work for your lifestyle.

- Avoid eating a large meal late in the evening, as it can affect digestion and sleep quality.

- Continue to be ingredient-aware – read the packaging! – when buying cans, yogurts and so on. (See page 15 for more on this and other long-term health tips.)

- Engage loved ones in your new lifestyle. Talk about your diagnosis and your journey and try recipes together.

- Portion control: be portion savvy.

- Plan ahead: prepare meals in advance.

- If you feel the urge to snack, pause and ask yourself, 'Am I really hungry, or just bored?' Could you find a displacement activity to distract you, such as gardening, walking, reading, colouring, painting or phoning a friend?

- With the 1-2-3 plan, snacking between meals is not recommended, but I understand that sometimes life happens and, where essential, snacking fills the void.

Eggs

A versatile, nutrient-dense power food, eggs are a complete high-quality protein source loaded with vitamins, minerals and good fats and are very low in carbs, too. They will keep you satisfied for longer, so you won't be reaching for that between-meal sweet treat. They are brilliant for breakfast, lunch, dinner or an occasional snack; there really isn't a wrong time to eat them.

You can enjoy eggs scrambled, in omelettes, fried, poached, boiled, in frittatas, quiches or as mini muffin omelettes. When cooking eggs, it is best to cook them low and slow, in butter.

Muffin omelettes

A great way to use up any leftover veg or ham at the end of the week is to make mini muffin omelettes. Finely chop up low-starch vegetables (tomatoes, courgettes, mushrooms and spring onions work well, or for a list of more low-starch veg, see page 78) and pop them in a bowl with 6–8 eggs. Whisk the eggs, add a pinch of salt and pepper, pour into mini muffin moulds and bake in an oven preheated to 180°C (350°F), Gas Mark 4 for 20 minutes until firm and domed. They make a great bite for lunch, with some salad.

Omelettes

With basic ingredients and a simple method, you can always add your own twist to an omelette. You just can't knock them from a nutrition, convenience and sustenance point of view, and even younger children can be taught to make them (with supervision).

The great thing about omelettes is that you can fill them with sweet or savoury ingredients, eat them warm, cold or rolled up to have on the go. You can serve them laid out flat, folded in half or cut into finger-length rolls. You can make them more fun and versatile when cooking for a family by lining up different fillings for people to choose from.

Omelette-making tips

- Always buy the best-quality eggs you can afford. Try to buy free-range and organic where possible.

- Use unsalted butter to cook them in, rather than margarine or any other oils.

- Beat the eggs well in a bowl or jug before pouring them into the pan. Make sure there are no flecks of white and the mixture is completely combined.

- If you can, use a nonstick heavy-based frying pan and make sure the butter is fully melted before you pour in the eggs.

- Low and slow heat wins the omelette race. Do not under- or overcook an omelette; you want to cook it over a medium-low heat and slowly, so the egg doesn't burn.

A SIMPLE OMELETTE

SERVES
1

PREP TIME
2 MINS

COOK TIME
7 MINS

3 eggs

unsalted butter

sea salt and cracked black pepper

NET CARBS	0G
FIBRE	0G
PROTEIN	23G
FAT	25G
KCAL	314

People make omelettes in a variety of ways, many of which are far too complicated. There is no need for milk, cream or water! If you are not a cook, but would like to make one thing well, then follow my simple steps for creating the perfect omelette.

1 Crack the eggs into a bowl and whisk until smooth. Season with salt and pepper.

2 Place a nonstick frying pan over a medium heat and melt a generous knob of butter.

3 Once the butter has melted and starts to sizzle, immediately pour in the egg mixture.

4 Using a spatula, carefully drag the outer edges of the omelette, where it is starting to stick, into the middle of the pan. Fill any gaps in the egg mix by tilting the pan from side to side. Do this a couple of times, until the mixture is noticeably starting to set.

5 Cook for 2–3 minutes, then carefully fold the omelette in half using the spatula and slide it on to a plate.

APPLE AND CINNAMON OMELETTE

SERVES
1

PREP TIME
5 MINS

COOK TIME
15 MINS

½ teaspoon coconut oil

60g (2¼oz) apple, cored and cut into
small cubes

20ml (1½ tablespoons) water,
plus more if needed

1 teaspoon ground cinnamon

3 eggs, lightly beaten

To serve

Greek yogurt

flaxseeds / linseeds, or pumpkin
seeds (optional)

NET CARBS	7.7G
FIBRE	1.9G
PROTEIN	23G
FAT	19G
KCAL	295

Have you ever tried a sweet omelette? If not, then this is a must. This flavoursome, protein-packed breakfast is incredibly filling and contains the scrumptious natural sweetness of apple and cinnamon.

1 Place a nonstick frying pan that has a lid over a medium heat and add the coconut oil. Once melted, place the apple into the frying pan with the measured water. Bring to the boil, then reduce the heat to a simmer. Pop on the lid and cook until the apple is soft (about 10 minutes). If the pan seems a little dry, splash in a bit more water.

2 Once the apple is soft, add the ground cinnamon and stir. Remove half of it to a bowl.

3 Pour the egg mixture into the pan and, using a spatula, carefully drag the outer edges of the omelette – where it is starting to stick – into the middle of the pan. Fill in any gaps in the egg mix by tilting the pan from side to side. Do this a couple of times until the mixture is starting to set.

4 Add the remaining apple and reduce the heat to low. Cook for 2–3 minutes before carefully folding the omelette in half using the spatula and sliding it on to a plate.

5 Serve immediately with a dollop of Greek yogurt. You could scatter over a few flaxseeds or pumpkin seeds, if you like.

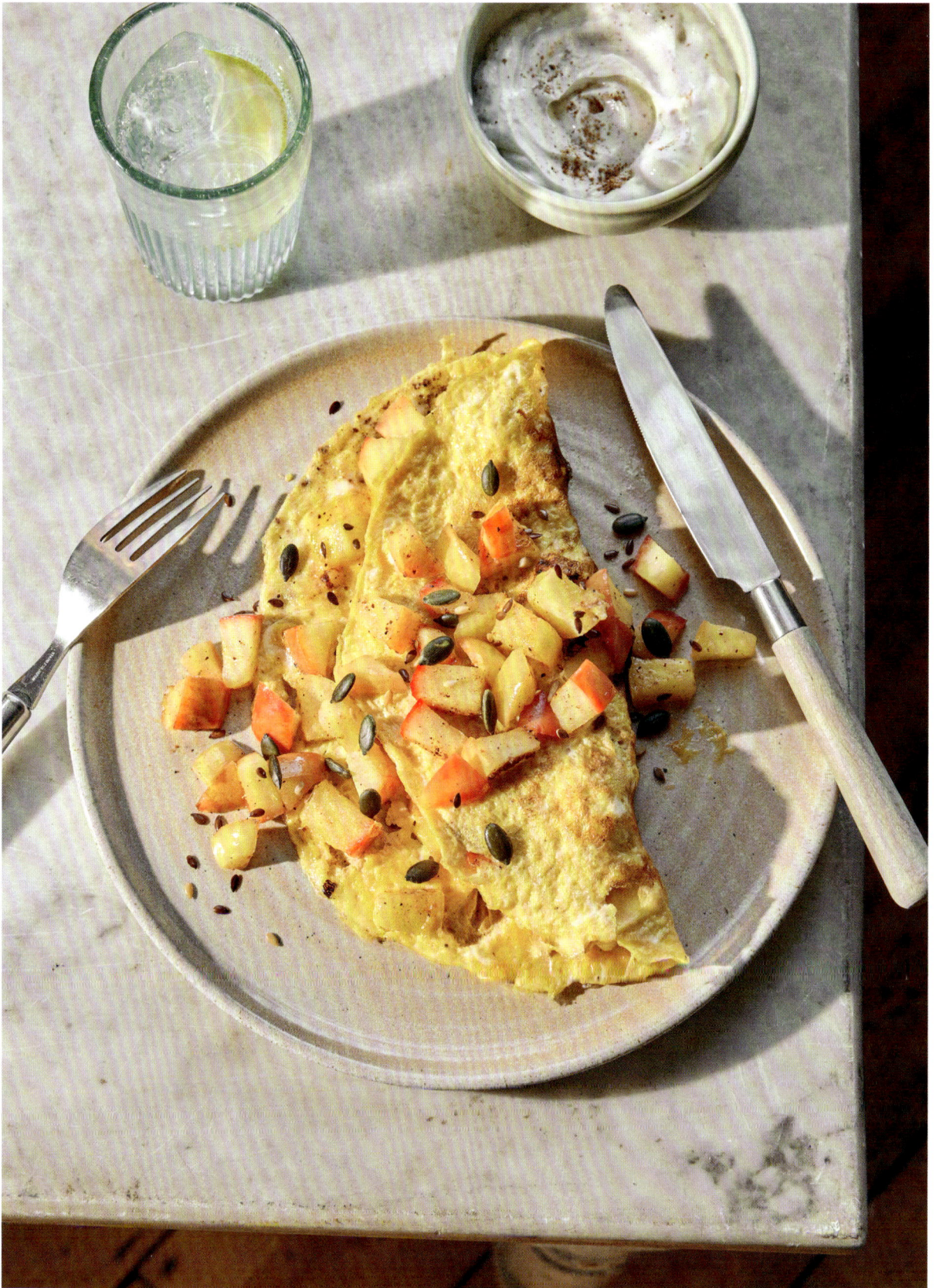

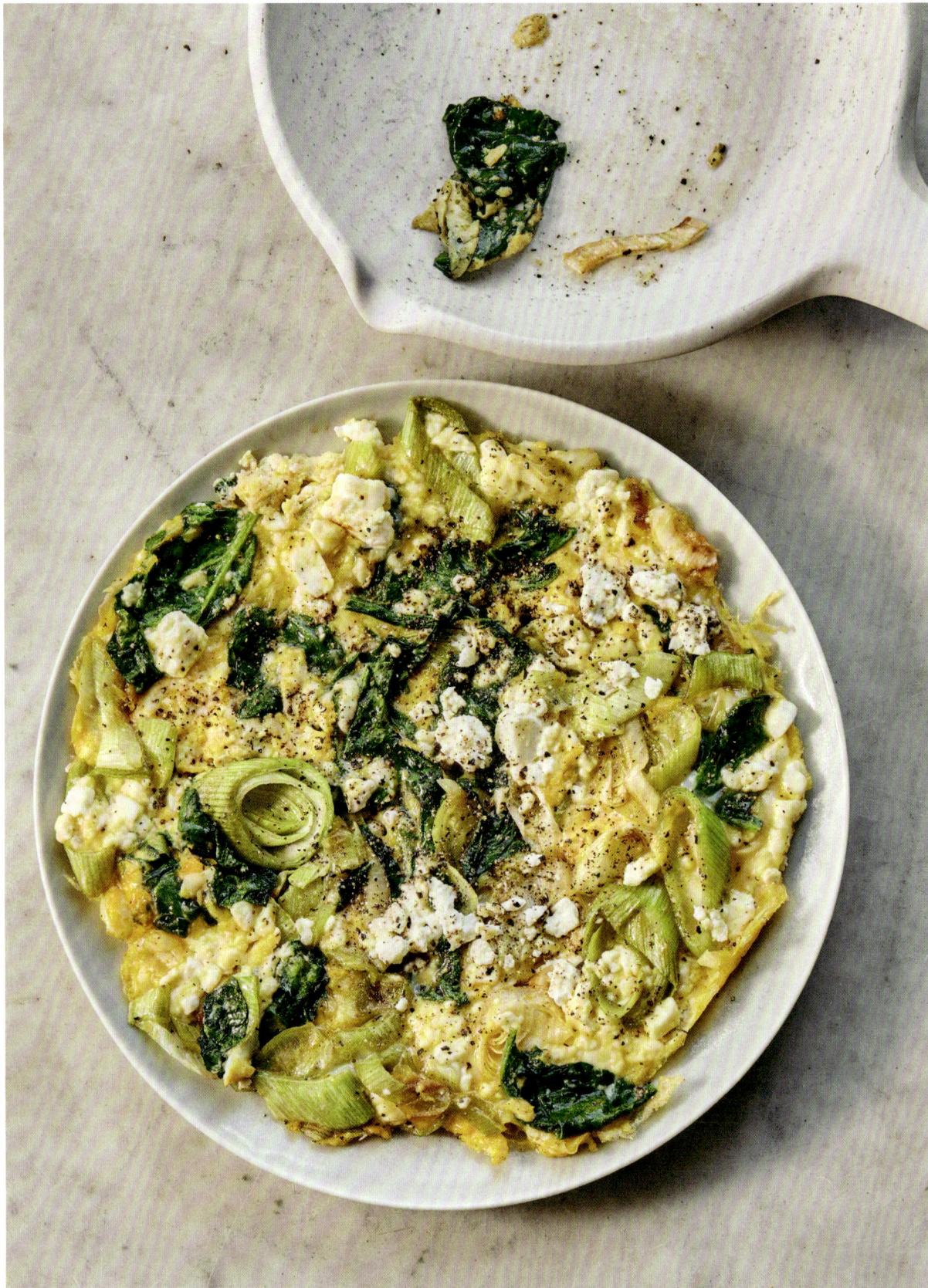

SPINACH, LEEK AND FETA OMELETTE

SERVES
1

PREP TIME
2 MINS

COOK TIME
15 MINS

1 tablespoon unsalted butter

80g (2¾oz) leek, finely sliced

2 handfuls of spinach

3 eggs, lightly beaten

30g (1oz) feta cheese, crumbled

sea salt flakes

NET CARBS	3.8G
FIBRE	2.6G
PROTEIN	30G
FAT	35G
KCAL	456

Leeks are a low-starch vegetable with a mild sweet onion flavour that pairs beautifully with the saltiness of feta. Of course, you may find your blood sugars react better to a savoury start, though this could be enjoyed for lunch or a light dinner, too. Protein-rich and filling, it is truly delicious.

1   Place a nonstick frying pan over a medium heat and add the butter. Once melted, add the leek. Once the leek has softened and started to caramelize, add the spinach. When the spinach leaves have wilted, pour in the eggs.

2   Using a spatula, carefully drag the outer edges of the omelette – where it is starting to stick – into the middle of the pan. Fill in any gaps in the egg mix by tilting the pan from side to side. Do this a couple of times until the mixture is starting to set.

3   Scatter over the crumbled feta and lightly season with salt to taste. Cook for 2–3 minutes before carefully folding the omelette in half using the spatula and sliding it on to a plate to serve.

PERFECT SOFT-BOILED 'JAMMY' EGGS
WITH CHILLI AND ALMOND BUTTER

SERVES
3

6 large eggs

4 teaspoons smooth 100 per cent almond butter

2 teaspoons chilli flakes

sea salt flakes

PER SERVING	
NET CARBS	0.9G
FIBRE	2.1G
PROTEIN	18G
FAT	18G
KCAL	241

PREP TIME
LESS THAN
5 MINUTES

COOK TIME
6 MINS

Eggs are a versatile nutritional powerhouse that provide you with so much goodness. They just need a little bit of love, a few added flavours, a little seasoning and to be cooked correctly. Follow these simple directions and you'll achieve perfection every time.

Try boiling six eggs every couple of days, allow them to cool and then pop them into the refrigerator inside an airtight container. This ensures you have an easy, quick, protein-rich, low-carb snack readily available.

1 Cook the eggs in a saucepan of boiling water for 6 minutes (medium-sized eggs take 5 minutes; small eggs take 4 minutes). Plunge into a large bowl or sink of cold water to prevent further cooking. Drain and leave to cool, then peel.

2 Cut in half, drizzle with almond butter and scatter with chilli and salt flakes.

RECIPE TIP

If you would like something to dip into your jammy eggs, a few asparagus spears (woody ends removed) make an excellent dipping choice. Place the spears into a pan of boiling water for 3–5 minutes until tender, but still vibrantly green.

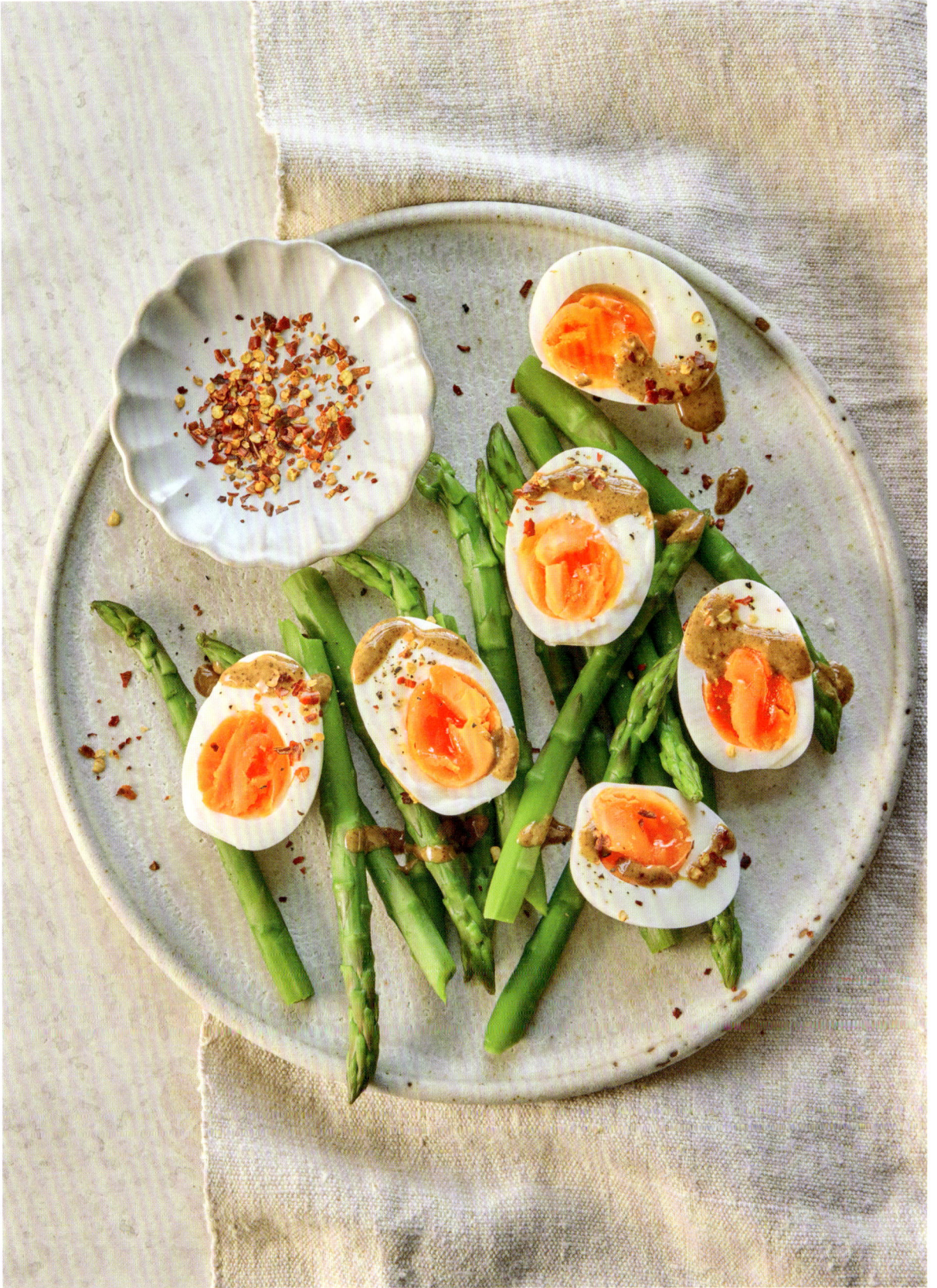

FLUFFY PANCAKES, BOTH SWEET 'N' SAVOURY

SERVES
3 / MAKES 6

PREP TIME
10 MINS

COOK TIME
5 MINS

2 large eggs

20g (¾oz) granulated sweetener

1 teaspoon baking powder

60g (2¼oz) Greek yogurt

20g (¾oz) arrowroot, coconut flour
  or gluten-free plain flour

2 teaspoons coconut oil

2 tablespoons water

FOR 2 PANCAKES	
NET CARBS	7.2G
FIBRE	0G
PROTEIN	6.4G
FAT	8.2G
KCAL	128

These are *incredibly* fluffy and an absolute crowd-pleaser. Serve as a sweet dish with berries and Greek yogurt or, for a savoury twist, try some fried shallots and cherry tomatoes with soured cream and chives.

1 Carefully separate the eggs. Place the whites in a scrupulously clean metal bowl (or they will be hard to whisk) and the yolks in another mixing bowl. Set the yolks aside.

2 Whisk the egg whites to stiff peaks, either by hand or with an electric whisk. Set aside.

3 Add the granulated sweetener to the yolks with the baking powder and Greek yogurt, whisking to achieve a light frothy consistency. Add the arrowroot (or sift in the flour) and combine to make a batter.

4 Using a silicone spatula, fold in the egg whites, little by little, until all the mixture is combined but still aerated, taking care not to over-mix.

5 Place a nonstick frying pan (ideally one that has a lid) over a medium heat. Add the coconut oil and melt. Once the oil is melted and hot, carefully add 2 dessertspoons of batter to the pan to make a pancake. (You may be able to cook 3 pancakes in the pan together.) Allow the undersides to cook: this will take 2–3 minutes. Make sure the heat is on medium as you do NOT want it to burn. Once the underside is cooked, you will be able to slide a spatula underneath it to flip it over.

6 Now add the 2 tablespoons of water to the pan, reduce the heat to medium-low and place a lid or large plate on top to allow the pancakes to steam for 2 minutes. This will ensure they are cooked through.

7 Continue cooking pancakes until all your batter has been used, then serve with berries and Greek yogurt.

RECIPE TIP
For a savoury twist, replace the granulated sweetener with 1 teaspoon dried parsley, 1 teaspoon dried chives, ½ teaspoon onion powder, ½ teaspoon salt and some pepper. Serve with fried shallots or tomatoes, 2 teaspoons soured cream and some finely chopped chives.

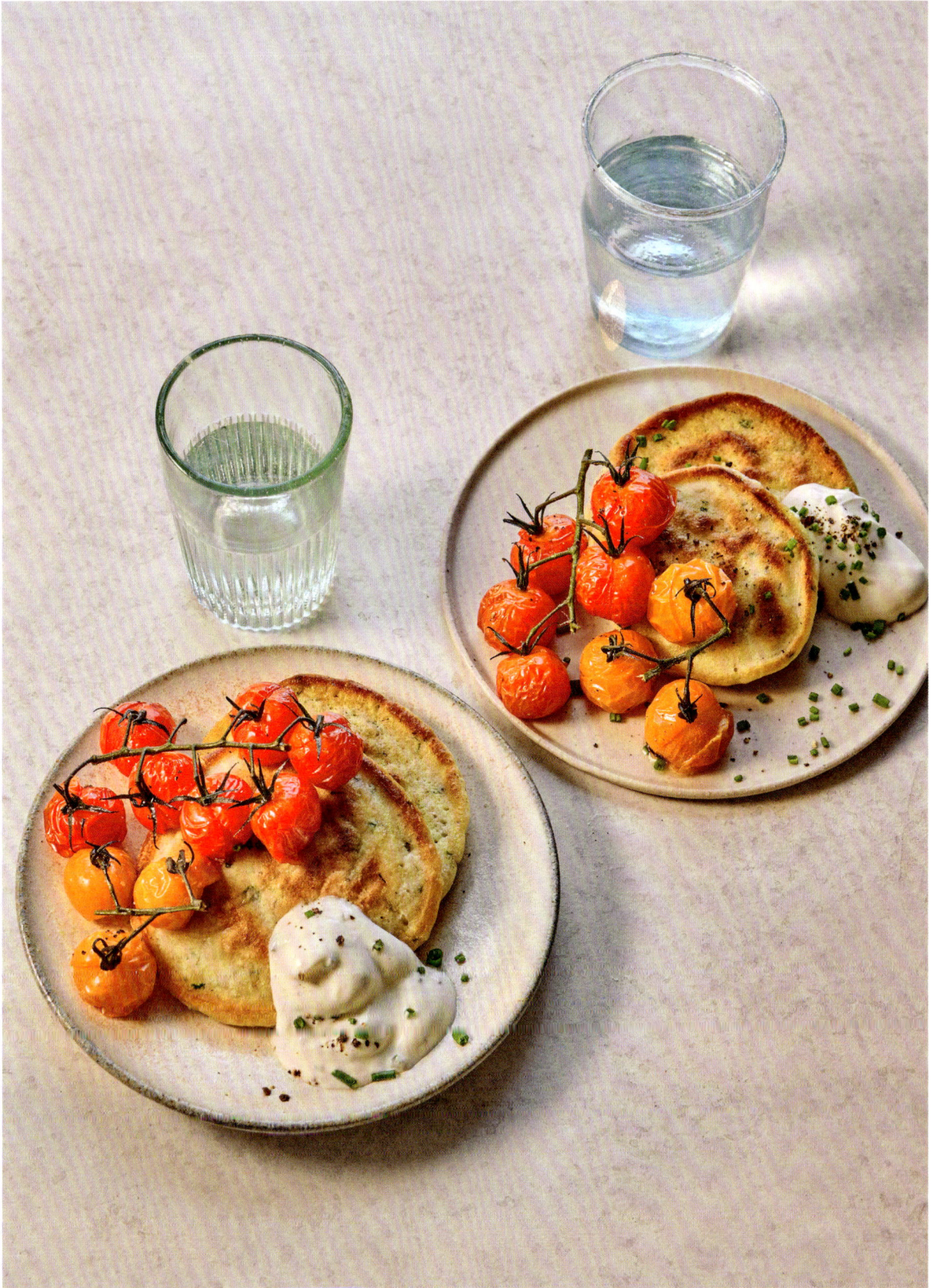

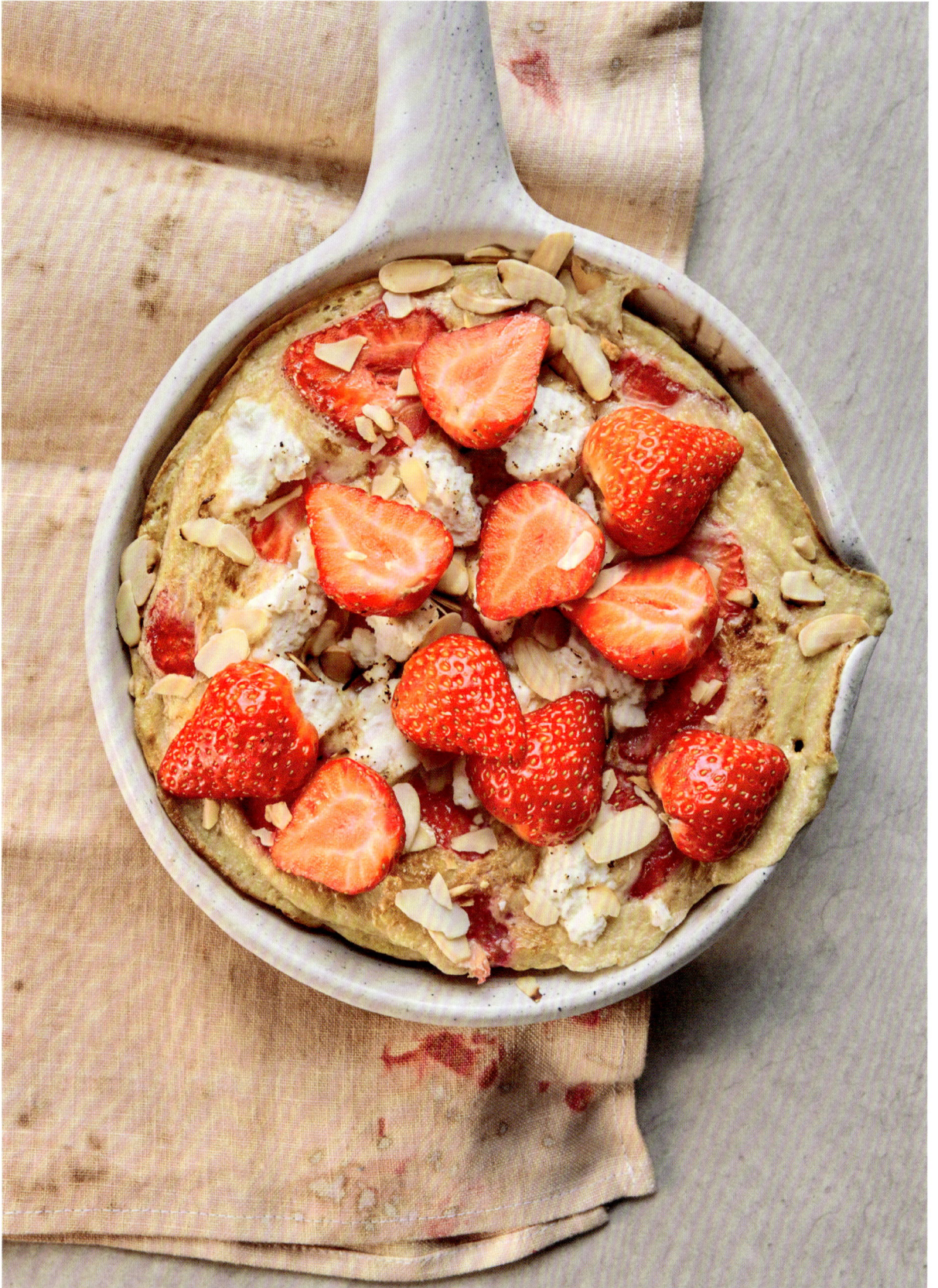

SWEET STRAWBERRY AND ALMOND FRITTATA

SERVES
4

PREP TIME
10 MINS

COOK TIME
12 MINS

250g (9oz) strawberries

2 tablespoons powdered sweetener

6 large eggs

50g ground almonds, or ground flaxseeds / linseeds

4 teaspoons sugar-free vanilla extract

10g (¼oz) unsalted butter

100g (3½oz) firm ricotta cheese, crumbled

40g (1½oz) toasted flaked almonds

PER SERVING	
NET CARBS	5.3G
FIBRE	4.6G
PROTEIN	17G
FAT	23G
KCAL	307

A delightful frittata that satisfies a sweet tooth and which you can slice and serve. This is a great source of protein and perfect for sharing with your family and friends.

If you're wondering what it tastes like, I tested the recipe on my four-year-old daughter and her best friend. Later that evening, I received a message from the best friend's mum asking what I'd cooked for them, as her daughter had described it as a 'delicious strawberry cookie toast cake'. A few mint leaves on top would make a beautiful garnish and turn it into a table centrepiece.

1   Hull and finely slice 150g (5½oz) of the strawberries, then set aside. Halve the remaining 100g (3½oz) strawberries.

2   Combine the halved strawberries with 1 tablespoon of the sweetener and 1 teaspoon of water in a bowl and stir.

3   Place the eggs, ground almonds, vanilla and the remaining 1 tablespoon sweetener into a separate bowl and whisk well until combined.

4   Preheat your grill to high.

5   Melt the butter in a nonstick ovenproof frying pan over a medium heat. Add the egg mixture and move it around for 30 seconds until it starts to stick. Top with the sliced strawberries, ricotta and half the flaked almonds. Leave for 4–5 minutes until the underside is cooked; you will know it's ready when you are able to lift the sides up slightly.

6   Now place under the grill for about 6 minutes until the ricotta is lightly browned and the mixture has set.

7   Carefully remove from the grill, top with the halved strawberries and remaining flaked almonds, slice and serve. Any leftovers will keep in the refrigerator in an airtight container for up to 3 days.

PERFECT CRÊPES

SERVES
2

PREP TIME
5 MINS

COOK TIME
10 MINS

unsalted butter or olive oil spray

110g (3¾oz) Greek yogurt

2 large eggs

40ml (2½ tablespoons) unsweetened almond milk, or other milk

25g (1oz) arrowroot

20g (¾oz) milled seeds or ground almonds

PER SERVING	
NET CARBS	14G
FIBRE	1.1G
PROTEIN	13G
FAT	21G
KCAL	300

If you adore crêpes (thin pancakes), but, like me, the regular variety just leaves your blood sugar pointing northwards, then this recipe will make your heart sing. It took many tests to create a recipe for perfect pancakes and you couldn't get anything closer to the real deal in taste and texture. And the best thing: these won't spike your blood sugars! They are perfect for a weekend breakfast to share with family or a loved one, and children adore them. Fill them with berries and Greek yogurt, or lemon juice and powdered sweetener. Or you could roll a savoury filling, such as cooked minced beef, inside them and top with crumbled ricotta and parsley. However you choose to enjoy them, I hope you will love them as much as I do.

1 Place the butter or a light spray of olive oil into a deep frying pan over a medium heat.

2 Put all the remaining ingredients in a mixing bowl and whisk together.

3 Ladle a little of the batter into the centre of a pan, using the bottom of the ladle to even out into a wafer-thin circular shape. Cook one side for 1–2 minutes.

4 Once it starts lifting and you can easily insert a spatula underneath it, you can turn it over to cook the other side.

5 Fill and serve. These can be enjoyed either hot or cold.

RECIPE TIP

Alternatives to the arrowroot for this recipe are gluten-free plain flour or buckwheat flour.

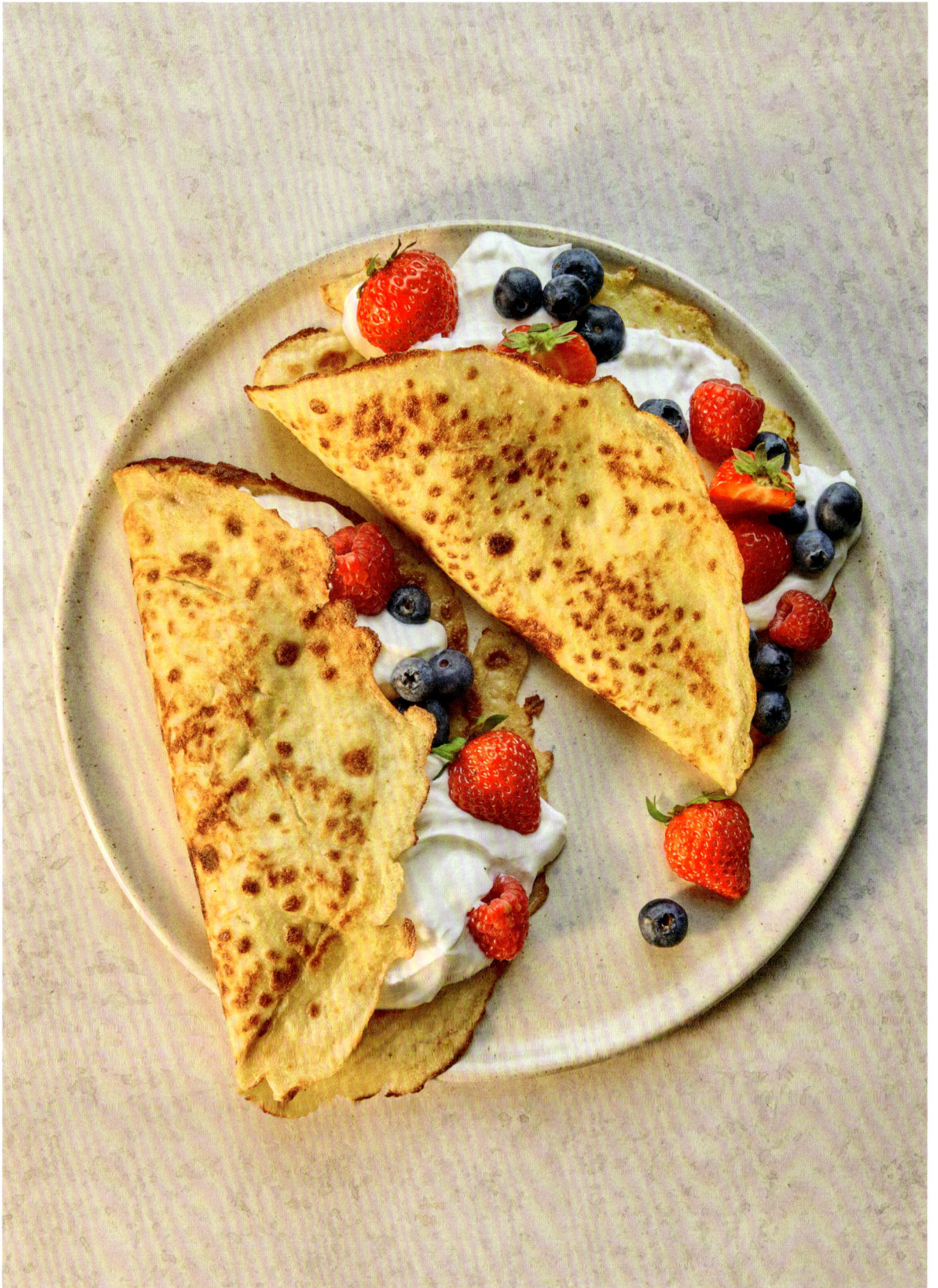

BAKED COURGETTE WRAP

SERVES
2

PREP TIME
10 MINS

COOK TIME
15 MINS

1 large courgette (300g / 10½oz)

6 large eggs

1 spring onion, finely sliced

2 tablespoons (15g / ½oz) arrowroot (optional)

1 tablespoon ground almonds

sea salt flakes and freshly ground black pepper

PER SERVING	
NET CARBS	10G
FIBRE	1.4G
PROTEIN	26G
FAT	20G
KCAL	325

Before my diabetes diagnosis, lunch used to be a shop-bought soup, a wrap and a low-fat fruit yogurt, foods I assumed were healthy choices. But they are packed with added sugars and salt and were fuelling my weight gain and lack of blood sugar control. This courgette roll is the perfect wrap alternative. It is easy to make and, once cooled, you can fill it with your favourite ingredients (try roasted red pepper and ricotta, Roasted Beetroot Hummus (see page 71) with spinach and feta, or chicken, light mayo, chopped lettuce and tomato.

1 Preheat the oven to 190°C (375°F), Gas Mark 5.

2 Coarsely grate the courgette and place it in a sieve lined with a sheet of muslin or a clean tea towel. Bring the corners of the cloth together and, holding the ends tightly, wring out any excess water from the courgette.

3 Lightly beat the eggs, salt and pepper in a bowl. Fold in the courgette, spring onion, arrowroot, if using, and ground almonds. Mix until you have a well-combined batter. Leave to stand for a few minutes to settle.

4 Pour the batter into an A4 paper-sized rectangle on a silicon-based baking sheet or reusable baking mat, making sure it is evenly spread out.

5 Bake for 15 minutes until firm, golden and cooked. Remove from the oven and leave it to cool.

6 Top with your favourite fillings.

RECIPE TIP

Parmesan would be a lovely addition to the base; add 30g (1oz) finely grated cheese to the batter at the same time as you fold in the grated courgette. For a spinach wrap, place 80g (2¾oz) spinach, 2 large eggs and 15g (½oz) arrowroot or gluten-free plain flour in a blender with salt and pepper and blend until it forms a bright green batter, then follow the method from step 4.

ONE-PAN BAKED EGGS
WITH VEGETABLES

SERVES
2 (OR SEE RECIPE INTRODUCTION)

PREP TIME
10 MINS

COOK TIME
15 MINS

1 teaspoon coconut oil, or unsalted butter

200g (7oz) carrot, coarsely grated

200g (7oz) red onion, finely chopped

1 garlic clove, finely chopped

3 handfuls of kale, coarse stalks removed, chopped

juice of ½ lime, or lemon

4 large eggs

sea salt flakes and cracked black pepper

small handful of chopped fresh coriander leaves, to serve

PER SERVING	
NET CARBS	16G
FIBRE	7.2G
PROTEIN	19G
FAT	14G
KCAL	284

One of those recipes that will stop all conversation around the table: everyone will sit in silence, totally hypnotized by the taste! This really is one of the best slice-and-share meals, being vibrant and packed with flavour and texture, as well as protein, essential vitamins and nutrients. Whether you are having this for breakfast, brunch, lunch or dinner, it is a total winner! It contains low-starch, fibre-rich veg to keep the calories and carbs low, while providing a filling meal.

This serves 2 hungry people, or it can be shared among 4 if you add smoked salmon and sliced avocado.

1 Melt the coconut oil or butter in a nonstick frying pan that has a lid and set over a medium-high heat. Add the grated carrot and fry for 2–3 minutes until it softens. Add the red onion and garlic and fry for a further few minutes until the onion softens and turns pale.

2 Add the kale and citrus juice, season with salt, then cook to soften the kale. As it wilts, keep moving the ingredients around the pan.

3 Crack an egg into each quadrant of the pan and add a generous twist of black pepper. Pop the lid on the pan and reduce the heat to medium-low. Cook until the whites have set (about 5 minutes).

4 Scatter with coriander and serve.

ONE-PAN VEGGIE BEAN BRUNCH
WITH EGGS

SERVES
2

PREP TIME
5 MINS

COOK TIME
20 MINS

1 teaspoon olive oil

400g (14oz) can of chopped tomatoes

2 tablespoons balsamic vinegar

2 teaspoons onion powder

1 tablespoon powdered sweetener

400g (14oz) can of cannellini beans,
   drained and rinsed

60ml (4 tablespoons) water

2 handfuls of spinach

4 large eggs

sea salt flakes

fresh coriander leaves, to serve
   (optional)

PER SERVING	
NET CARBS	38G
FIBRE	10G
PROTEIN	29G
FAT	17G
KCAL	449

Saturday mornings can be a little chaotic in our house: both my daughters have clubs, so we are faced with a list of chores and places to be. Come mid-morning we can be ravenous and this is where this recipe comes into its own: we all sit down to eat it together and it is a really good kick-starter for the weekend. Really easy to make, this is a nutritious take on baked beans using simple ingredients and you could eat it for any meal, it doesn't just have to be brunch. If you add chopped-up sausage with the cannellini beans, it becomes a sausage hotpot of sorts.

1 Put a drizzle of olive oil into a large frying pan and set over a high heat. Once hot, add the tomatoes and bring to the boil for a few minutes.

2 Pour in the balsamic vinegar and continue to cook for a further 2 minutes until the mixture starts to thicken a little. It will develop a deeper red colour.

3 Next, add the onion powder and reduce the temperature to medium-low. The mixture will thicken. Continue to cook over a low heat for a further minute or so.

4 Now add the sweetener and salt to taste, mix through, then add the beans and the measured water. Bring to the boil over a high heat. Cook for 5 minutes or so, stirring regularly so that nothing sticks.

5 Stir through the spinach and allow it to wilt into the bean mixture. Stir for a minute or so before reducing the heat to medium-low.

6 Crack an egg into each quadrant of the pan and slowly cook until the whites are set: this will take 7–10 minutes over a medium-low heat. You do not want the beans to burn, so it is best to do this slowly, but you could place a lid over your pan, if you have one, to set the top of the eggs and speed the process up a little.

7 Remove from the heat and scatter with coriander leaves to serve, if you like.

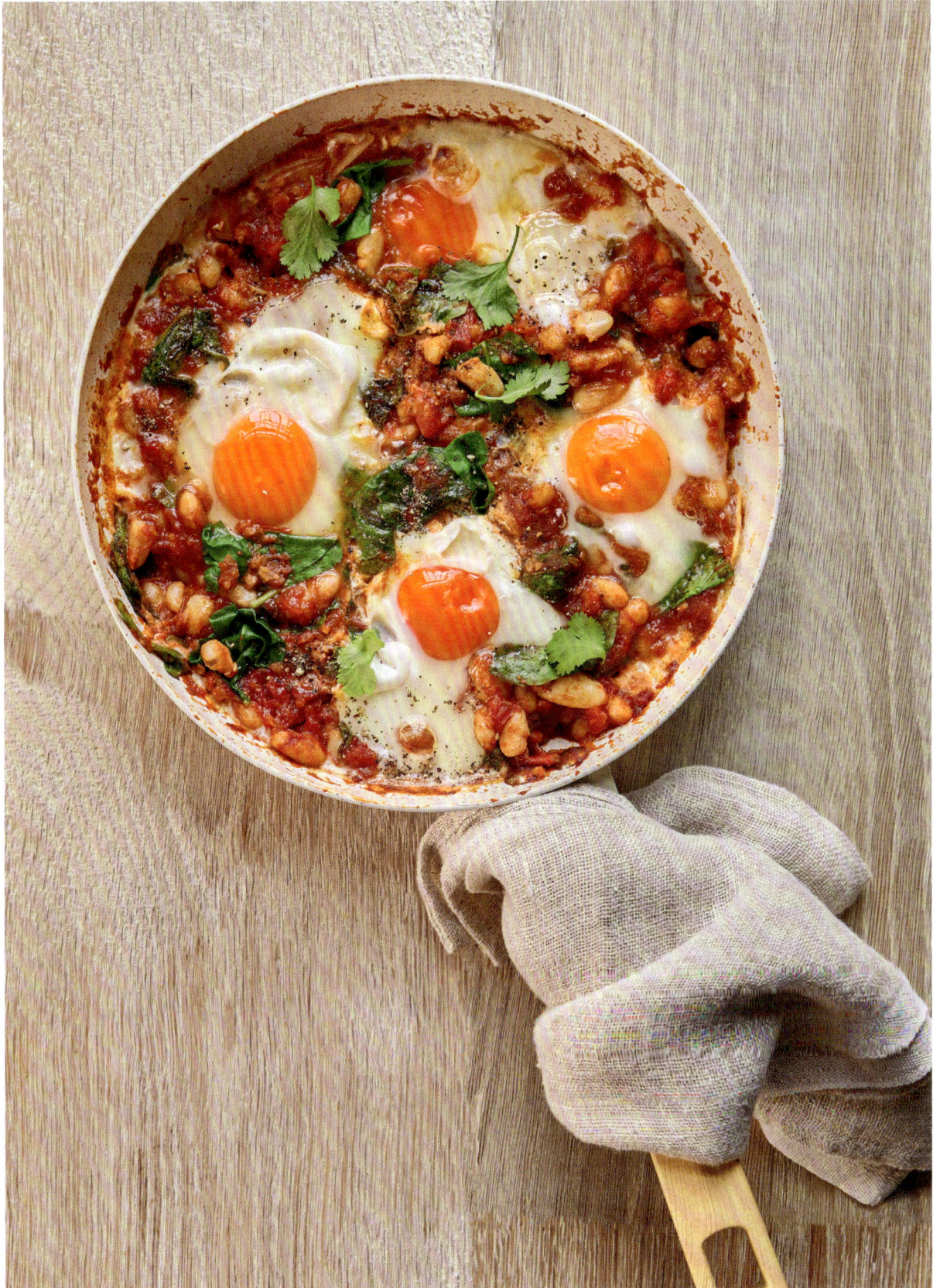

CHOCOLATE-PEANUT POT

SERVES

1

100g (3½oz) Greek yogurt

12g (½oz) crunchy 100 per cent peanut butter

5–10g (⅛–¼oz) powdered sweetener, such as erythritol (optional)

10g (¼oz) 70 per cent cocoa solids chocolate

1 teaspoon chopped unsalted peanuts, or 2–3 raspberries

NET CARBS	9.9G
FIBRE	2.3G
PROTEIN	9.8G
FAT	22G
KCAL	279

PREP TIME

10 MINS, PLUS CHILLING TIME

Tastes like a dessert in a pot… but without the added sugars, and this is also low in carbs and high in protein. These pots are perfect for breakfast or a snack and are easy to make in minutes the night before you need them. It's important not to ban tasty ingredients, but to understand how to use them in a measured way, so you still get to enjoy them. Peanut butter is very high in calories, so only use a small amount. Using a high cocoa content chocolate will keep the carbs low, reducing any blood sugar spike and maintaining balanced blood sugars.

1   Place the yogurt, peanut butter and sweetener, if using, into a ramekin or small bowl and stir, then smooth it out so the surface is even, ready for the chocolate to lay on top.

2   Melt your chocolate (for the method, see page 185), pour over the top of the yogurt mixture and smooth it out.

3   Add a few chopped peanuts or the raspberries.

4   Place in the refrigerator to set for at least 5 minutes or up to overnight.

RECIPE TIP   Choose a peanut butter with 100 per cent peanuts and no additives. Avoid peanut butters with added oils, salts and sugars.

'CARROT CAKE BATTER' OVERNIGHT OATS

SERVES

1

15g (½oz) organic jumbo oats

30g (1oz) carrot, grated, plus more (optional) for the top

10g (¼oz) chia seeds, plus more (optional) for the top

2 teaspoons powdered sweetener

½ teaspoon ground cinnamon

¼ teaspoon ground allspice

10g (¼oz) ground flaxseeds / linseeds

1 teaspoon sugar-free vanilla extract

120ml (4fl oz) unsweetened almond milk

For the topping

1 teaspoon cream cheese

2 teaspoons thick Greek yogurt

2 teaspoons powdered sweetener, plus more if needed

1 walnut, chopped (optional)

NET CARBS	14G
FIBRE	9.1G
PROTEIN	7.8G
FAT	16G
KCAL	246

PREP TIME

15 MINS,
PLUS OVERNIGHT CHILLING

A prep-ahead, grab-and-go breakfast, thick, creamy and delicious. High in fibre and protein, this is a tempting pot that tastes like a decadent dessert. Living with diabetes, oats can be a challenging ingredient, as they can spike blood sugars. However, they are fantastic if you can achieve the correct balance. In this recipe you use a small amount, which means they add a dose of fibre and lots of creamy texture. This is a breakfast that's easy to transport to the office or eat on the go.

1 Place the oats, grated carrot, chia seeds, sweetener, cinnamon, allspice and flaxseeds in a bowl and mix together. Now add the vanilla and almond milk. Mix together until all the ingredients are combined, then transfer to a jar or small bowl.

2 For the topping, place the cream cheese, Greek yogurt and powdered sweetener in a small bowl, mix together and taste. Add a little more sweetener if required.

3 Carefully spoon the cream cheese mix on top of the carrot batter and smooth it out with the back of a spoon. Add a few chopped walnuts or some more grated carrot or chia seeds for decoration. Cover and place in the refrigerator overnight.

RECIPE TIP

I use a natural powdered sweetener (erythritol) as it contains zero carbs and zero calories. Should you choose to use a sugar, such as honey or maple syrup, then please adjust the nutritional information accordingly, especially if you're living with diabetes or are insulin-dependent. If you would rather omit the oats, consider replacing them with ground flaxseeds / linseeds.

OVERNIGHT BERRY POTS

SERVES

4

PREP TIME

15 MINS, PLUS CHILLING TIME

COOK TIME

6–8 MINS

250g (9oz) strawberries, chopped

150g (5½oz) raspberries

4 tablespoons water, plus more if needed

3 tablespoons powdered sweetener, such as erythritol

200g (7oz) Greek yogurt

1 teaspoon sugar-free vanilla extract

2 tablespoons unsalted butter

60g (2¼oz) ground flaxseed / linseed

40g (1½oz) desiccated coconut

½ teaspoon ground cinnamon

PER SERVING	
NET CARBS	8.8G
FIBRE	9.6G
PROTEIN	5.9G
FAT	24G
KCAL	302

A no-bake, triple-layer pot that will inspire you to leap out of bed and rush towards the refrigerator to tuck into breakfast! This is full of healthy fats, vitamins, fibre and protein.

1 Place the chopped strawberries, raspberries and measured water in a small saucepan and set over a medium heat. Bring to the boil, then cook until the fruit has softened (6–8 minutes). You might need to add a little more water to stop the fruit from sticking to the pan.

2 Once the fruit has softened, gradually add the sweetener, tasting as you go. Once it is at the correct sweetness for you, pour it into 4 glass serving jars or bowls.

3 Mix the Greek yogurt and vanilla in a separate bowl, then spoon on top of each portion of strawberries and raspberries.

4 Place the butter, ground flaxseed, desiccated coconut and cinnamon in a small clean saucepan and set over a medium-low heat. Mix thoroughly until the butter is melted and you have achieved a biscuit crumb-like consistency. Spoon the mix on top of each portion.

5 Put into the refrigerator for at least 1 hour or up to overnight, until ready to serve.

RECIPE TIP You could use rhubarb instead of berries, cooked in the same way, for a spring seasonal option.

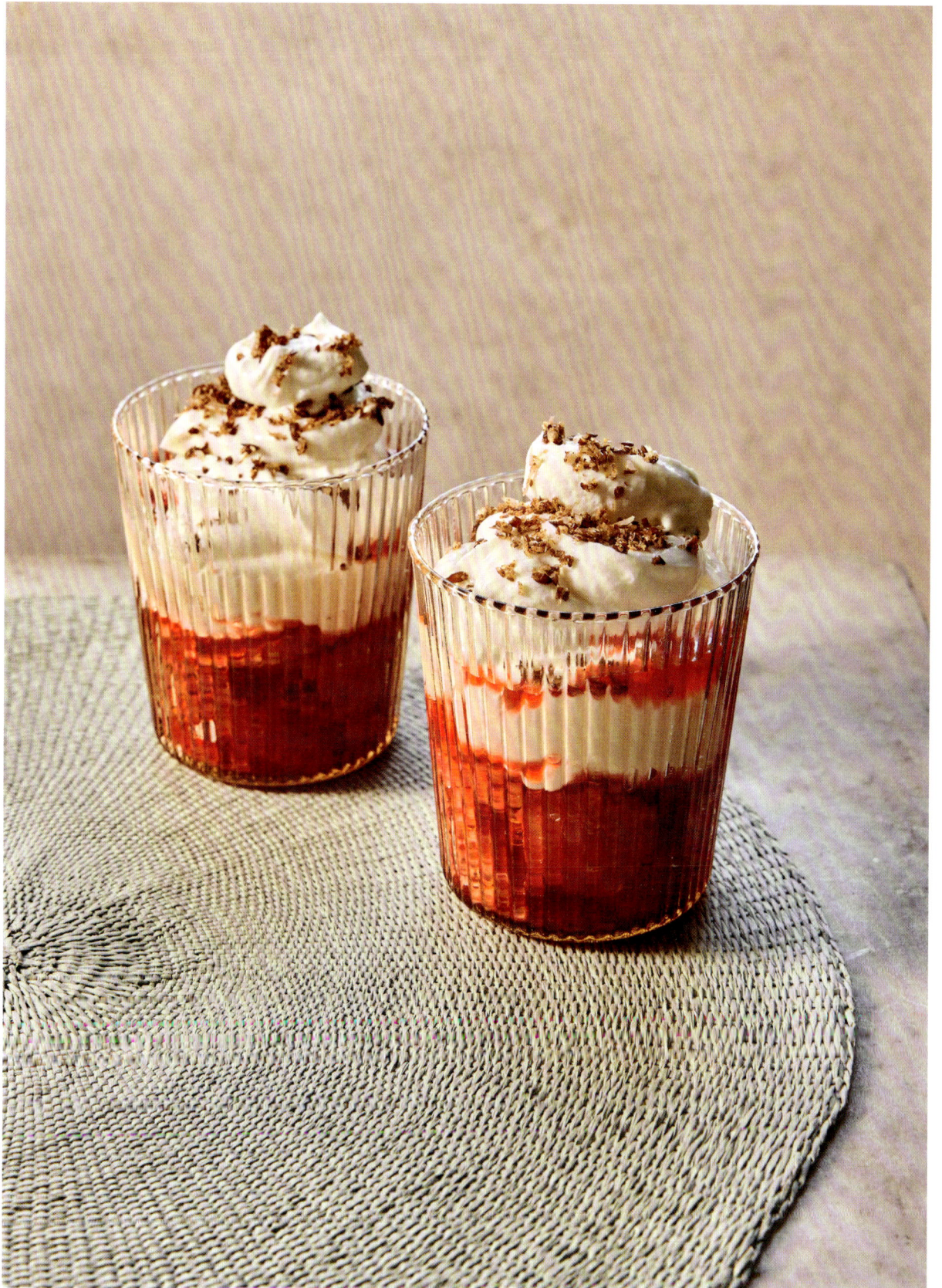

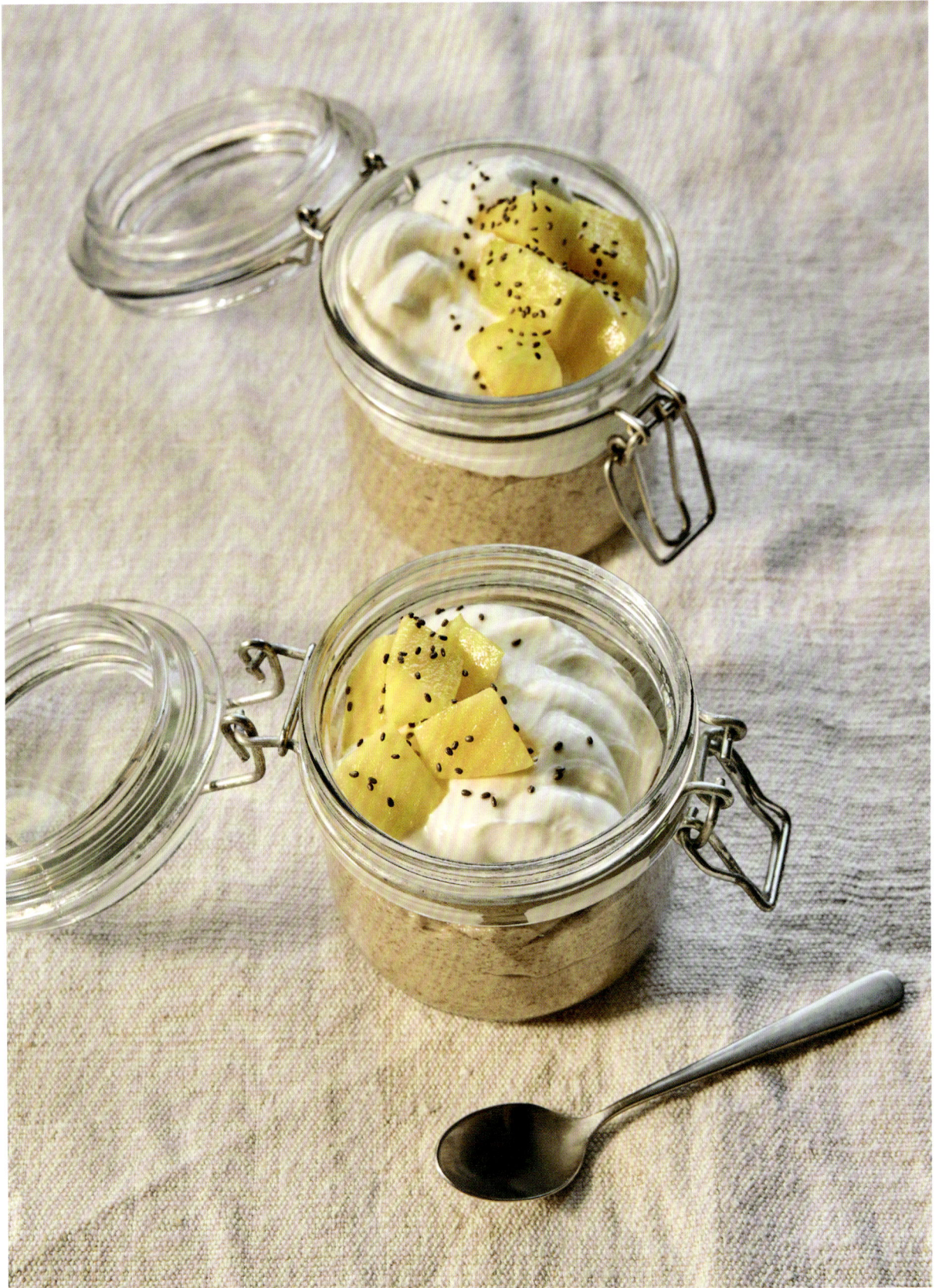

MANGO, COCONUT AND CHIA POTS

SERVES
2

PREP TIME
5 MINS, PLUS CHILLING TIME

For the base

40g (1½oz) oats or ground flaxseeds / linseeds

100g (3½oz) mango, plus more (optional) to top

15g (½oz) chia seeds, plus more (optional) to top

100ml (3½fl oz) canned coconut milk

100ml (3½fl oz) unsweetened almond milk

For the topping

60g (2¼oz) Greek yogurt

20ml (4 teaspoons) canned coconut milk

sugar-free vanilla extract, to taste

If you can tolerate oats and are able to enjoy them in a small, manageable portion, then this convenient, quick breakfast might just be perfect for you. You can prepare it the night before and have it ready to put in your bag and take to work. The combination of oats and chia create a wonderful creamy texture, while the mango and coconut add a tropical taste.

1 To make the base, put the oats, mango, chia, coconut milk and almond milk into a blender. Blend to achieve a custard-type consistency (it will thicken later). Pour into 2 small jars or ramekins.

2 Place the Greek yogurt, coconut milk and vanilla in a small bowl. Mix together well and spoon on top of each mango pot.

3 Top with chia seeds or some chopped mango and place in the refrigerator for 1 hour, or overnight.

PER SERVING	
NET CARBS	22G
FIBRE	5.3G
PROTEIN	7G
FAT	18G
KCAL	289

BREAKFAST AND BRUNCH

PEPPERY PARMESAN COURGETTE FRIES

SERVES
2

PREP TIME
10 MINS

COOK TIME
25 MINS

1 large courgette

1 large egg

50g (1¾oz) finely grated Parmesan cheese

30g (1oz) ground almonds

sea salt flakes and freshly ground black pepper

PER SERVING	
NET CARBS	5G
FIBRE	2.2G
PROTEIN	18G
FAT	19G
KCAL	265

VEGETARIAN

A great alternative to potato fries and a fantastic side dish or occasional snack. These also work well dipped in boiled eggs, a nutritious alternative to toast (see Jammy Eggs with Chilli and Almond Butter, page 96).

1 Preheat the oven to 200°C (400°F), Gas Mark 6. Line a baking sheet with nonstick baking paper.

2 Cut off the top and bottom of the courgette, then cut it in half down its length and finally slice it into fries.

3 Crack the egg into a shallow bowl and lightly beat. Place the Parmesan, ground almonds and a generous pinch of salt and pepper in another shallow bowl, mix together and flatten out.

4 Take a courgette baton and coat it in the egg, then roll it in the Parmesan crumbs. Place on the prepared baking sheet. Repeat the process until all the batons are covered in crumbs.

5 Roast in the oven for 15 minutes, then use a spatula to flip them over carefully and cook for a further 10 minutes until golden brown.

6 Remove from the oven and allow to cool for a few minutes before plating up.

RECIPE TIP You could serve these with one of my Dips 4 ways (see pages 68–71).

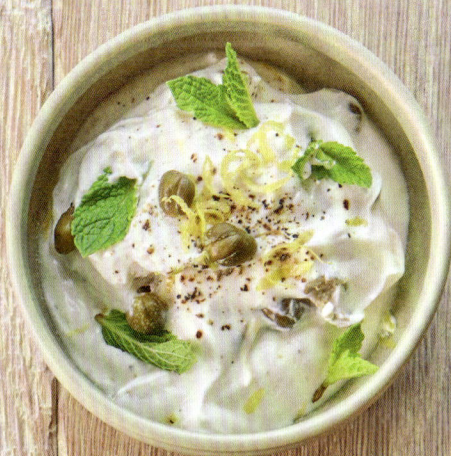

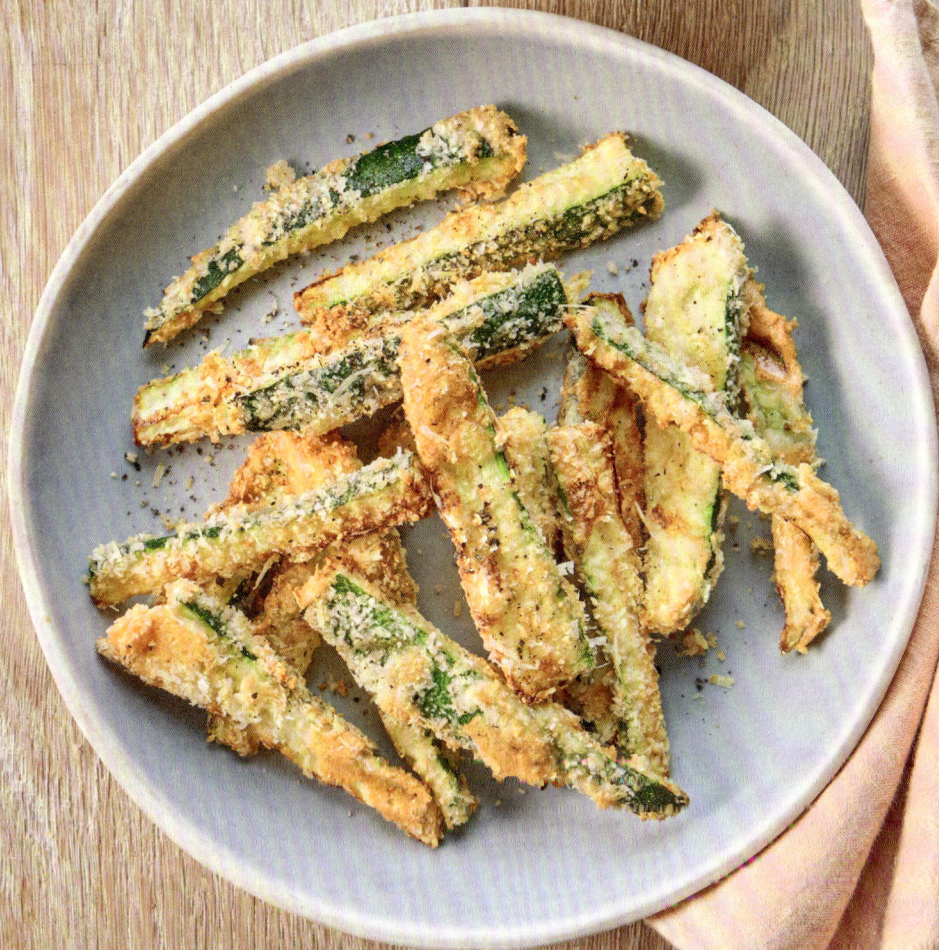

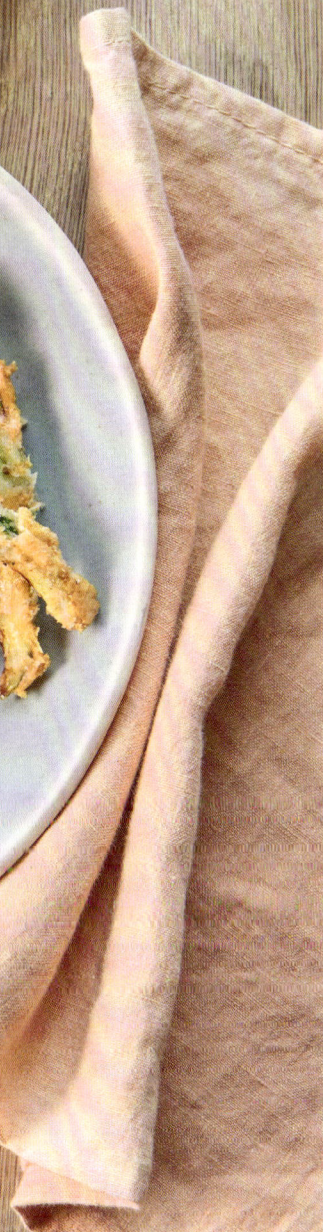

ROASTED BUTTERNUT
WITH BROCCOLI PESTO

SERVES
2

PREP TIME
15 MINS

COOK TIME
45 MINS

1 butternut squash (about 1kg / 2lb 4oz), halved and seeds scooped out

olive oil spray

1 teaspoon sea salt flakes

seeds from ½ pomegranate

1 tablespoon capers

freshly ground black pepper

For the pesto

100g (3½oz) broccoli

10 Brazil nuts

4 tablespoons olive oil

15g (½oz) basil leaves

PER SERVING	
NET CARBS	35G
FIBRE	11G
PROTEIN	9.9G
FAT	41G
KCAL	573

A feast for the eyes: you'll be wanting to photograph and share this! It is so vibrant and colourful and it packs a nutritional punch, too. The sweetness of the squash alongside the deep flavours of the pesto are a match made in food heaven. This is a filling dish and it works well for lunch or dinner.

The pesto recipe here makes enough to fill a small jar and is sufficient to use for several meals.

1 Preheat the oven to 170°C (340°F), Gas Mark 3½.

2 Place the squash halves flesh-side up on a baking sheet. Lightly spray with oil and season with the salt and a pinch of pepper. Roast for about 45 minutes until you can easily push a fork into them, and the flesh has started to brown and peel away from the skin.

3 For the pesto, put all the ingredients into a food processor with a pinch of salt and 1 teaspoon of pepper and blend. You will probably have to use a spatula to scrape down the sides until smooth and combined. Add a little cold water, 1 tablespoon at a time, if the mix is not sufficiently smooth, and keep blending. Taste and adjust the seasoning if required.

4 Once the squash has been removed from the oven, spoon about 1 tablespoon of pesto on it and spread evenly until the whole surface is covered. Scatter with the pomegranate seeds and capers.

5 Serve immediately, or leave to cool and keep in an airtight container in the refrigerator. Eat within 3 days.

SPINACH AND RICOTTA STUFFED MUSHROOMS

SERVES

2

PREP TIME

10 MINS

COOK TIME

25 MINS

4 Portobello mushrooms

olive oil spray

60g (2¼oz) ricotta cheese

30g (1oz) spinach leaves, finely chopped

1 garlic clove, crushed

sea salt flakes and freshly ground black pepper

chilli oil, or 1 teaspoon finely chopped chives, to serve

PER SERVING	
NET CARBS	7.3G
FIBRE	2.4G
PROTEIN	14G
FAT	13G
KCAL	203

Brilliant with baked salmon for dinner, or smoked salmon for brunch. It is easy to make and could even be used as part of a packed lunch.

1 Preheat the oven to 180°C (350°F), Gas Mark 4.

2 Carefully remove the stalks from the Portobello mushrooms. Finely chop the stalks.

3 Spray olive oil into a large ovenproof baking dish and add the Portobello mushroom caps, stalk-sides up. Spray with olive oil.

4 Place the ricotta, spinach and garlic in a bowl with the finely chopped mushroom stalks and season with salt and pepper. Spoon the mixture evenly between the mushroom caps, then bake for 20–25 minutes until the ricotta is golden brown and the mushrooms are cooked.

5 Serve hot with a little drizzle of chilli oil or scattered with chopped chives, or leave to cool and eat within 24 hours.

VEGETARIAN

RECIPE TIP

If you wish to add a little finely grated Parmesan, please do so, scatter it over 15 minutes before the end of baking. (Please note that this will change the nutritional information.)

ROASTED CRISPY MISO CHICKPEA AND PUMPKIN SALAD

VEGETARIAN

SERVES	PREP TIME	COOK TIME
2	20 MINS	1 HOUR

For the chickpeas

400g (14oz) can of chickpeas, drained

1 tablespoon olive oil or sesame oil

15g (1 tablespoon) miso paste

1 teaspoon smoked paprika

For the salad

200g (7oz) peeled and deseeded
   pumpkin or butternut squash,
   chopped into 4cm (½ inch) cubes

olive oil spray

3 large handfuls of spinach

1 large courgette

1 tablespoon finely chopped
   mint leaves

sea salt flakes and freshly ground
   black pepper

PER SERVING	
NET CARBS	40G
FIBRE	15G
PROTEIN	20G
FAT	13G
KCAL	389

RECIPE TIP

The crispy chickpeas are best stored at room temperature: leave to cool completely before placing in an airtight container. Eat within 3 days.

If you haven't tried roasting chickpeas before, I urge you to do so! They create a fabulous topping for a salad or a nutritious snack, they are fibre-rich and lower in calories than nuts and seeds, but still crunchy and flavoursome, plus they provide a healthy dose of protein.

1 Preheat the oven to 180°C (350°F), Gas Mark 4. Line a baking sheet with nonstick baking paper.

2 Pop the chickpeas on kitchen paper and pat them dry: they need to be totally dry before cooking, or they won't crisp up.

3 Place the olive oil, miso paste and smoked paprika in a bowl and thoroughly mix together. Add the chickpeas and coat them with the other ingredients. Tip on to the prepared baking sheet and spread them out evenly.

4 Roast for 25–30 minutes until golden brown and fragrant, shaking the baking sheet halfway through to ensure all sides cook evenly. The longer you leave them in the oven, the crisper they will become. Remove from the oven.

5 Increase the oven temperature to 200°C (400°F), Gas Mark 6. Line a baking sheet with nonstick baking paper.

6 Place the pumpkin in a bowl, spray with olive oil, season with salt and pepper and lightly toss to coat. Spread on to the prepared baking sheet and bake for 20 minutes, then flip them over and bake for a further 10 minutes until tender with caramelized edges. Set aside.

7 Place the spinach in a bowl. Using a vegetable peeler, peel down the length of the courgette into ribbons. Once you reach the seeds, turn the courgette and repeat on the other side (discard or compost the seeds). Add the courgette ribbons to the bowl with the spinach, spray with olive oil and toss together with the mint.

8 Divide the mixture between 2 serving bowls. Top with the roast pumpkin and 3 tablespoons of the crispy chickpeas. Season to taste with salt and pepper before serving.

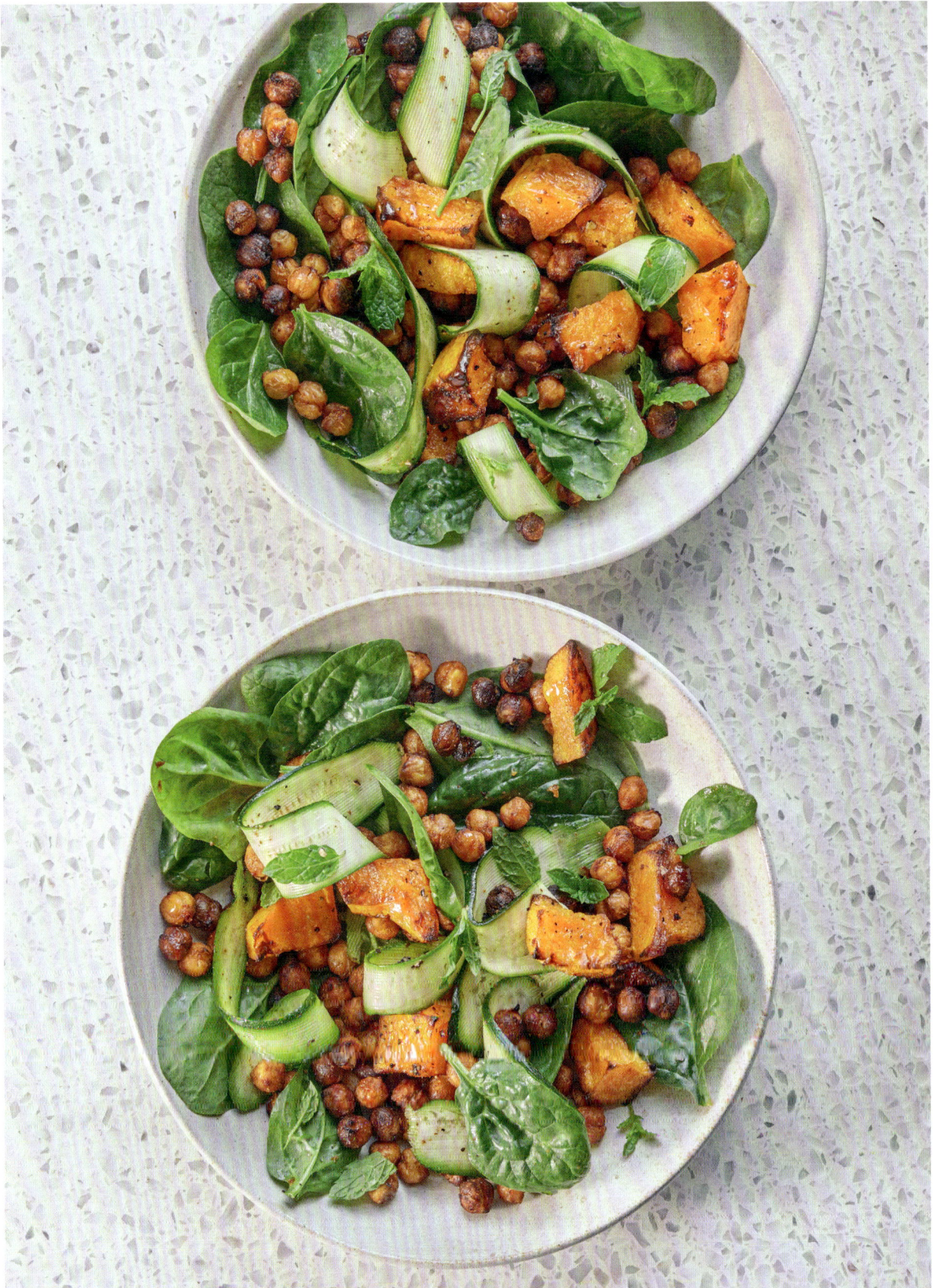

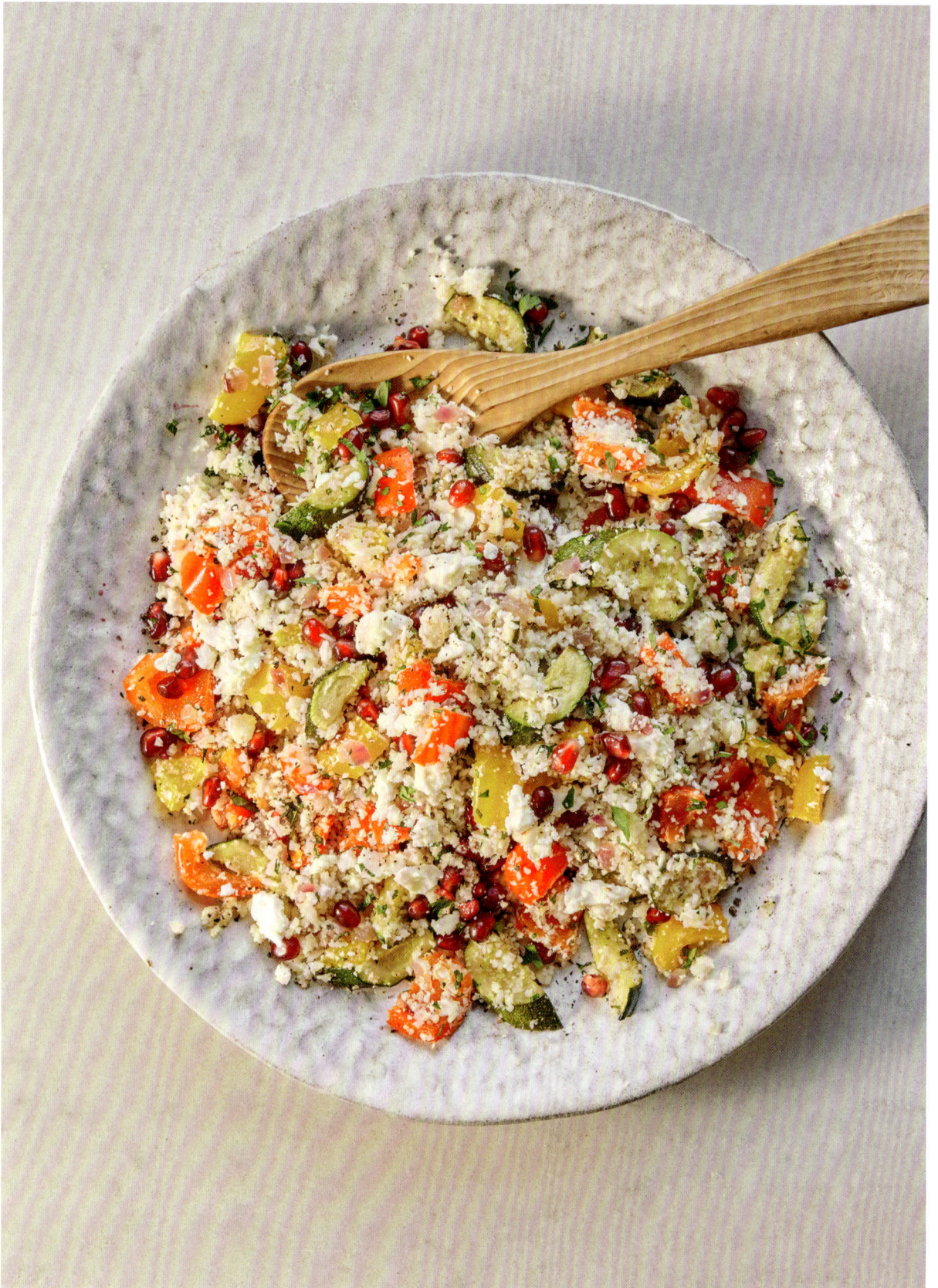

CAULIFLOWER 'COUSCOUS'
WITH ROASTED VEGETABLES

SERVES
6 AS A SIDE DISH,
OR 3 AS A MEAL ON ITS OWN

PREP TIME
15 MINS

COOK TIME
30 MINS

For the base

1 small red onion, finely chopped

1 red pepper, cut into bite-sized pieces

1 yellow pepper, cut into bite-sized
   pieces

1 small courgette, sliced

olive oil spray

1 cauliflower

2 tablespoons apple cider vinegar

seeds from ½ pomegranate

70g (2½oz) feta cheese, crumbled

1 tablespoon chopped mint leaves

1 tablespoon chopped flat leaf
   parsley leaves

sea salt flakes

PER SERVING (AS A SIDE)	
NET CARBS	13G
FIBRE	3.6G
PROTEIN	5.5G
FAT	3.5G
KCAL	110

This has a sweet and savoury element to it and is loaded with roasted vegetables. You won't believe how beautiful and vibrant a dish containing cauliflower can look, or that this doesn't contain any grains. It is full of fresh flavours and an interesting variety of textures, providing a perfect accompaniment to a piece of baked fish or a chicken skewer.

1 Preheat the oven to 180°C (350°F), Gas Mark 4.

2 Place the red onion, peppers and courgette in a bowl with a spray of olive oil and a generous pinch of sea salt. Massage the ingredients together, then tip on to a baking tray and bake for 30 minutes until soft and cooked. Shake occasionally to make sure nothing is sticking or burning.

3 Once cooked, tip into a serving bowl and leave to cool.

4 Meanwhile, roughly chop the cauliflower into small pieces. Put into a food processor along with the stalk and leaves, or grate with a grater. You want to achieve a couscous-like consistency.

5 Heat 1 tablespoon oil in a large saucepan over a medium heat. Add the cauliflower 'couscous' and a pinch of salt. Gently toast it for 1–2 minutes, stirring. Be careful not to overcook, as you want the pieces to be tender.

6 Toss the 'couscous' again and add to the serving bowl of roasted vegetables. Mix the apple cider vinegar in gently. Top with the pomegranate seeds, feta and herbs, then serve

7 Keep any leftovers in an airtight container in the refrigerator and eat within 24 hours.

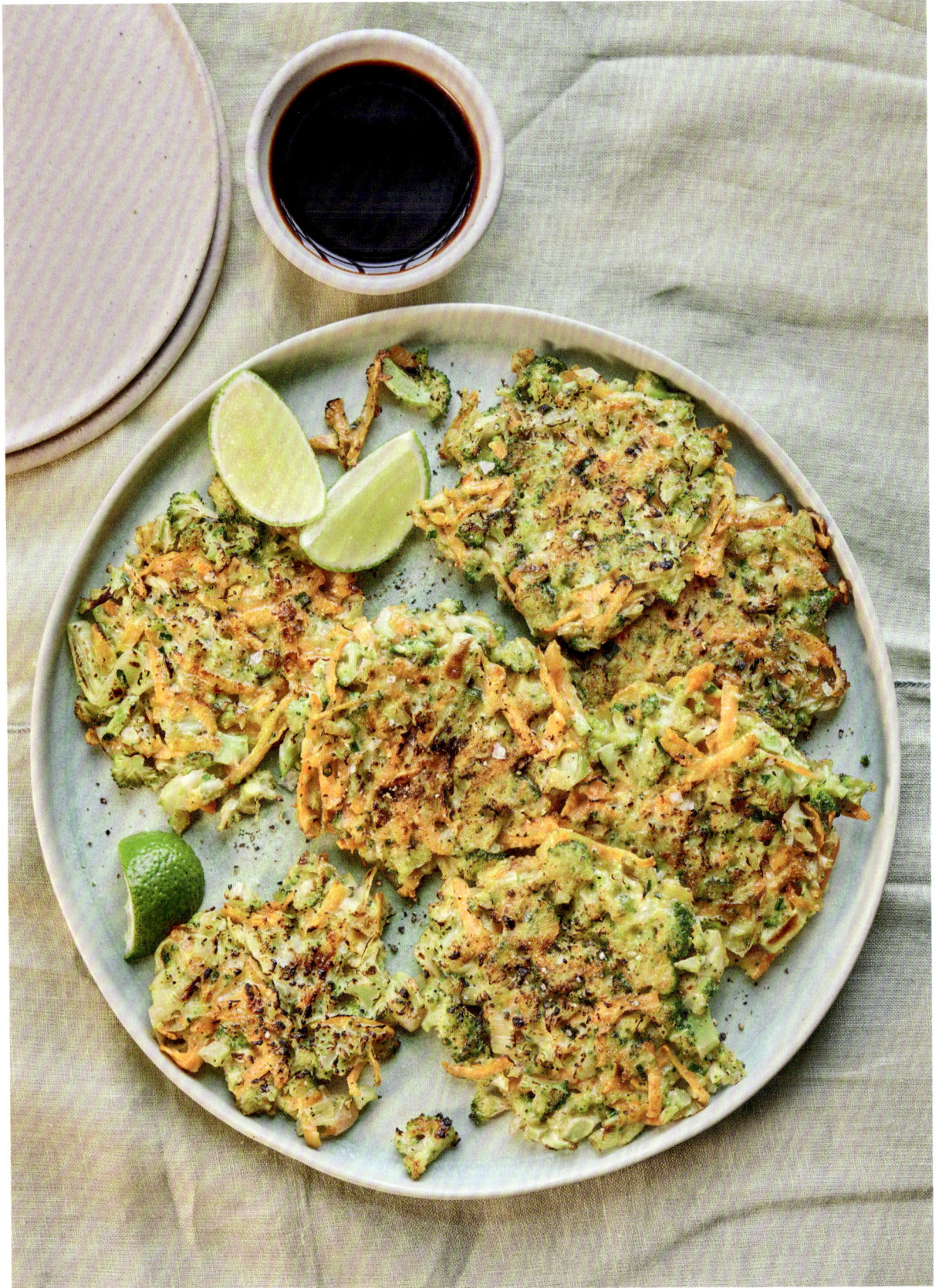

BROCCOLI, LEEK AND SWEET POTATO FRITTERS

SERVES
4/MAKES 8

PREP TIME
15 MINS

COOK TIME
10 MINS

150g (5½oz) broccoli

70g (2½oz) sweet potato

2 teaspoons unsalted butter

light olive oil spray

50g (1¾oz) leeks, sliced

2 teaspoons finely chopped chives

12g (½ oz) arrowroot

2 large eggs, lightly beaten

25ml (1fl oz) low-salt soy sauce (optional)

PER SERVING	
NET CARBS	8.6G
FIBRE	2.3G
PROTEIN	6G
FAT	7.6G
KCAL	131

This has a sweet and savoury element to it, and is loaded with roasted vegetables. You won't believe how beautiful and vibrant a dish containing cauliflower can look, or that this doesn't contain any grains. It is full of fresh flavours and an interesting variety of textures, providing a perfect accompaniment to a piece of baked fish, or a chicken skewer.

1 Place the broccoli on a chopping board, divide it into florets with a sharp knife, then finely chop into a rice-like consistency. Or place in a food processor and pulse-blend a few times. Tip into a bowl.

2 Peel the sweet potato and coarsely grate it into the broccoli bowl.

3 Melt 1 teaspoon of the butter and a light spray of olive oil in a frying pan over a high heat. Sauté the sliced leeks until soft and fragrant, then tip into the broccoli and sweet potato mix. Add the chives, arrowroot and eggs and mix to form a batter.

4 Clean your frying pan and place over a medium heat. Spray with olive oil and add the other 1 teaspoon butter. Place 1 heaped tablespoon of fritter batter into the pan and spread it out a little so it is about 2cm (¾ inch) thick; you may be able to fit 3–4 fritters in the pan at the same time.

5 Allow the underside to cook for 2–3 minutes until golden brown, then carefully flip over like a pancake. Allow the other side to cook for a further 2–3 minutes until golden brown. Repeat this process until you have used all the batter.

6 Serve straight from the pan, or allow to cool and serve cold. Serve with the soy sauce, if you like.

RECIPE TIP
It is best to fry leeks in a mixture of light olive oil and butter, as this results in a fabulous depth of flavour from the butter, while the olive oil helps to prevent the butter from burning.

VEGETARIAN

SMOKY SWEET POTATO FRIES

SERVES
2

PREP TIME
10 MINS

COOK TIME
25 MINS

olive oil spray

1 large sweet potato (350g/12oz), cut into fries

2 teaspoons smoked paprika

1 teaspoon garlic purée

sea salt flakes and freshly ground black pepper

PER SERVING	
NET CARBS	35.5G
FIBRE	5.5G
PROTEIN	2.5G
FAT	2.5G
KCAL	192

VEGETARIAN

Sweet potatoes are higher in calories and carbohydrates than many low-starch veg, so they should be enjoyed in moderation. A small handful can be added to a plate filled with salad or green vegetables and a good serving of protein. These fries are beautifully seasoned and tender inside, perfect for the whole family. They can be served with my Kale, Garlic and Avocado Cream (see page 68) or as a side dish to Marinated Chicken Kebabs or a homemade burger (see pages 157 and 150).

1 Preheat the oven to 190°C (375°F), Gas Mark 5. Spray a baking tray with a little olive oil, or line it with nonstick baking paper.

2 Place the fries in a large mixing bowl, spray them with olive oil and sprinkle with salt, pepper, the smoked paprika and garlic purée. Mix well to lightly coat all the fries.

3 Spread the fries evenly over the prepared baking tray and bake for 15 minutes. Carefully remove the tray from the oven, turn the fries over to ensure they cook evenly, then bake for a further 10 minutes until crispy with a soft centre.

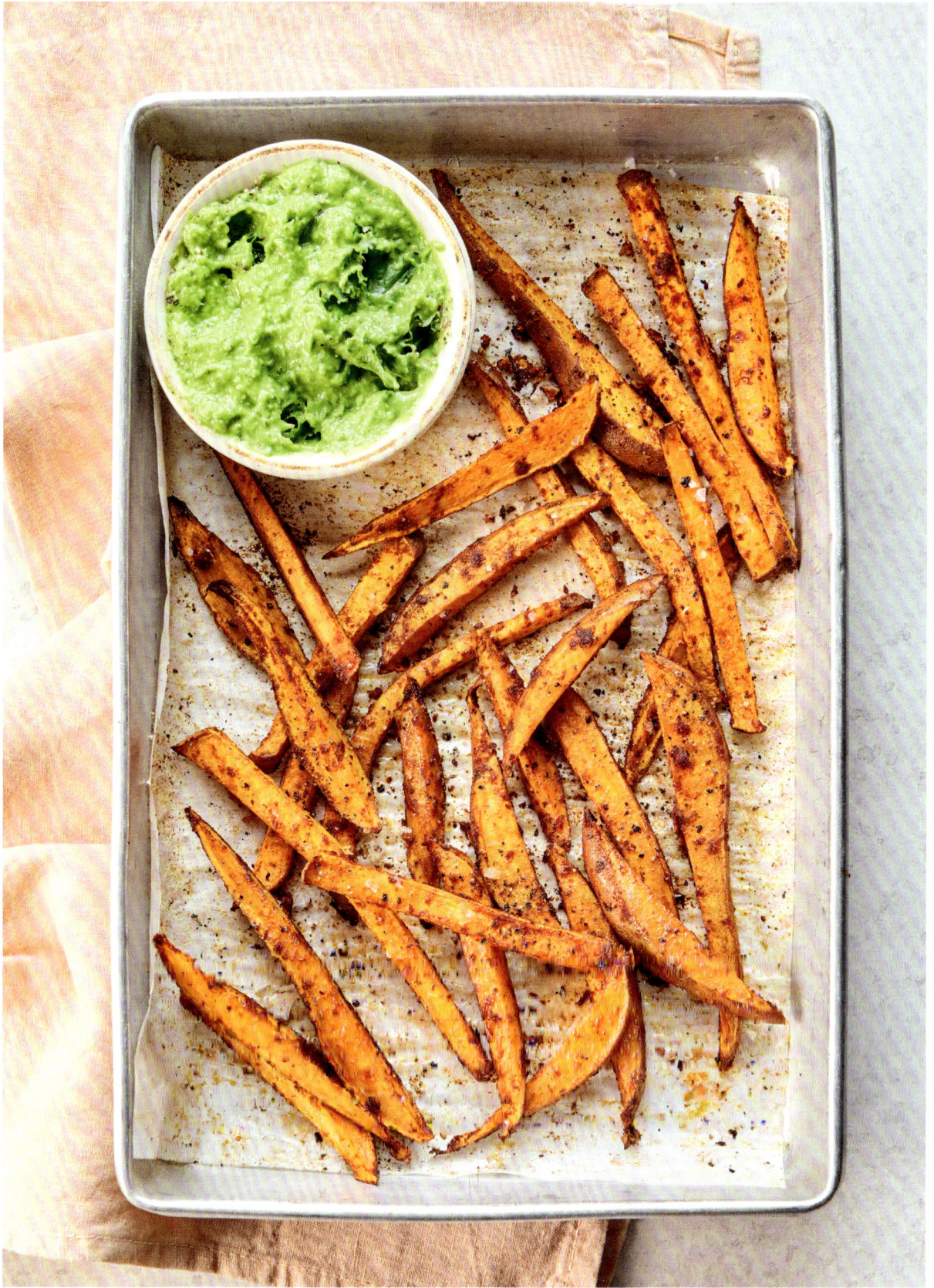

ROASTED PANEER AND TOMATO CURRY
WITH COCONUT CAULIFLOWER 'RICE'

SERVES
3

PREP TIME
20 MINS

COOK TIME
30 MINS

For the curry

225g (8oz) pack of paneer, cut into 2cm (¾ inch) cubes

olive oil

2 teaspoons ground cumin

1 teaspoon ground coriander

2 teaspoons garam masala

1 red onion, chopped

1 red pepper, finely chopped

1 teaspoon garlic purée, or 1 garlic clove, finely chopped

1 teaspoon ground turmeric

2 teaspoons sweetener

350g (12oz) fresh tomatoes, or a 400g (14oz) can of tomatoes

4 tablespoons water

4 tablespoons Greek yogurt

40g (1½oz) spinach, chopped

sea salt flakes and cracked black pepper

For the coconut cauliflower 'rice'

650g (1lb 7oz) cauliflower florets

2 teaspoons coconut oil

2 tablespoons desiccated coconut

½ teaspoon ground cumin

PER SERVING	
NET CARBS	32G
FIBRE	8.7G
PROTEIN	32G
FAT	36G
KCAL	598

Divine. There, I said it. This rich, thick and aromatic curry tastes as though it has been cooked for hours, but takes just 40 minutes to prepare.

1 Preheat the oven to 200°C (400°F), Gas Mark 6. Put the paneer in a bowl and season with salt and pepper. Spray with a light drizzle of olive oil and toss. Spread on a nonstick baking sheet in a single layer and cook for 20 minutes or until golden around the edges, then set aside to cool.

2 Meanwhile, heat a splash of olive oil in a large saucepan over a medium-high heat. Stir in the cumin, coriander and garam masala and cook until fragrant (about 2 minutes). Add the onion and red pepper and sauté for 5 minutes until soft. Stir in the garlic, turmeric, sweetener and a small pinch of salt. Cook for a further minute or so.

3 Stir the tomatoes and the water into the onion mixture. Break the tomatoes down with a wooden spoon. Reduce to a simmer and cook, stirring, for 5 minutes. Remove from the heat and add the mixture to a blender with the yogurt. Blend until smooth. Taste and season, if needed.

4 Add a spray of olive oil to the onion mixture and add the chopped spinach. Gently cook for a minute until it begins to wilt. Stir in the paneer, pour in the curry sauce and stir. Bring to the boil, then simmer until the consistency is thick and creamy.

5 Meanwhile, blitz the cauliflower florets in a food processor until you achieve a rice-like consistency (or use a box grater.) Place in a clean tea towel to drain any excess water..

6 Melt the coconut oil in a deep frying pan over a high heat. Add the cauliflower 'rice' and coconut and cook for a minute before adding the cumin and a pinch of salt. Cook for a further 3–4 minutes, stirring regularly to prevent sticking. Serve immediately with the curry on top.

RECIPE TIP
If paneer is not to your taste, substitute any other lean protein. If using chicken, add it to the sauce at the same time as the onion, but in this case, do not blend the sauce. If you do prefer a smoother sauce, you will have to remove the chicken before blending.

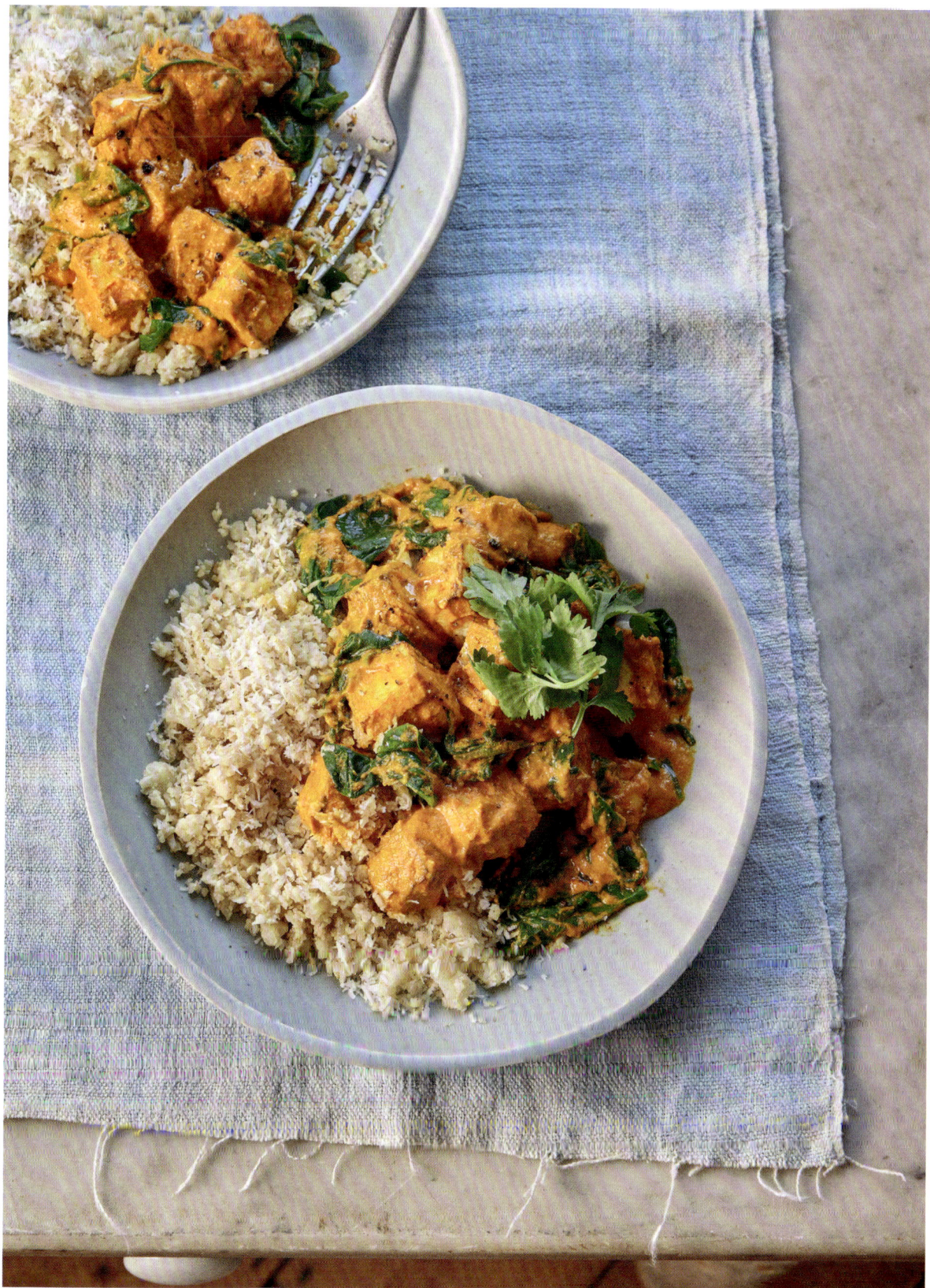

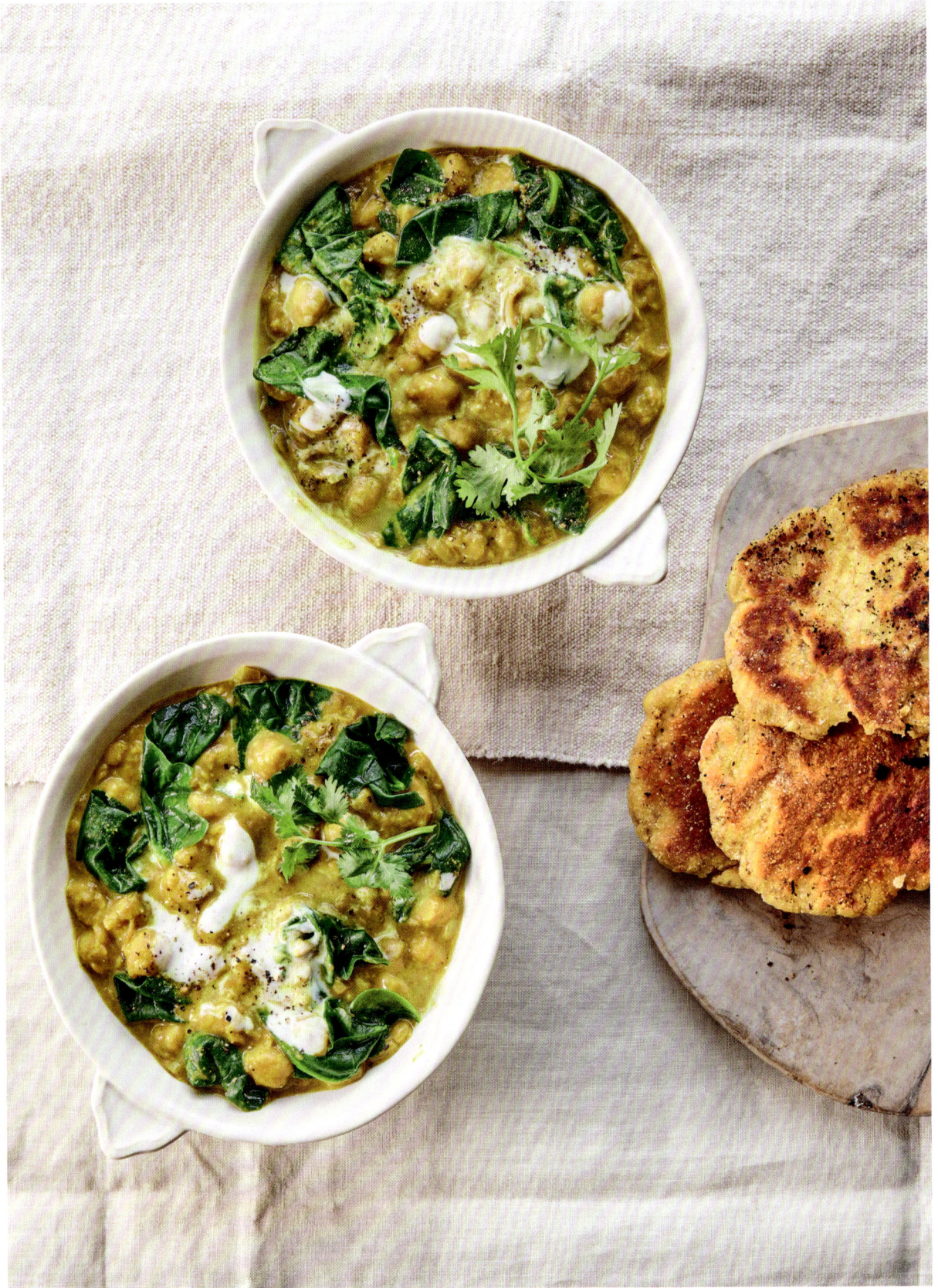

CHICKPEA DAL

SERVES
4

PREP TIME
10 MINS

COOK TIME
40 MINS

2 tablespoons olive oil

200g (7oz) onion, finely chopped

1 garlic clove, finely chopped

2 teaspoons ground cumin

2 teaspoons ground coriander

1 teaspoon ground turmeric

1 teaspoon ground ginger

3 tablespoons water

400ml (14fl oz) can of coconut milk

1 tablespoon smooth 100 per cent
   peanut butter

1 vegetable stock cube

400g (14oz) can of chickpeas, drained
   and rinsed

2 handfuls of spinach leaves

50ml (1¾fl oz) kefir, or 50g (1¾oz)
   Greek yogurt, plus more to serve

coriander, to serve

This is a nourishing, protein-rich, low-calorie meal that is full
of flavour. It is bright, vibrant and perfect to portion up and eat
throughout the week, or freeze it to use at a later date. It is a dish
which children will devour very happily, a proven indicator that it
is temptingly tasty! If you need an extra side dish, serve this with
roasted cauliflower, coconut cauliflower 'rice' (see page 126), or a small
portion (20g /¾oz) of quinoa.

1 Heat the olive oil in a wok or large frying pan. Once the oil is hot,
   add the onion and fry for about 6 minutes or until translucent with
   lightly browned edges. Add the garlic and fry for another minute
   or so until soft.

2 Add all the spices (cumin, coriander, turmeric and ginger) and stir
   into the onion mix with the measured water to create a fragrant paste.
   Fry for a couple of minutes before pouring in the coconut milk, peanut
   butter and stock cube. Thoroughly mix together and let the mixture
   bubble for a minute or so.

3 Tip in the chickpeas and stir thoroughly into the mixture. Bring to
   the boil, then reduce the heat to medium-low and simmer for about
   30 minutes. Stir the mixture regularly to ensure the chickpeas do not
   stick. You could try using a potato masher and mashing the mix a
   couple of times during cooking, so the chickpeas are broken down and
   help to thicken the sauce.

4 Stir in the spinach. Once it wilts, add the kefir or Greek yogurt. Serve in
   a bowl with a swirl of kefir or yogurt, scattered with chopped coriander.

PER SERVING	
NET CARBS	19G
FIBRE	6.1G
PROTEIN	9.1G
FAT	28G
KCAL	372

RECIPE TIP
Dal will keep in an airtight container in the refrigerator for
up to 5 days. It can be gently reheated on the hob or in the
microwave until it is piping hot. Or portion it up and freeze for
up to 3 months. To defrost, place in the refrigerator overnight
before reheating to piping hot.

VEGETARIAN

ROASTED VEGETABLE QUICHE
WITH A CHEDDAR CRUST

SERVES
4 / MAKES 8 SLICES

PREP TIME
10 MINS

COOK TIME
35 MINS, OR MORE IF YOU ARE
ROASTING VEGETABLES FRESH

For the filling

352g (12oz) roasted vegetables (or see below)

6 large eggs

3 tablespoons canned low-fat coconut milk

40g (1½oz) feta cheese, crumbled

freshly ground black pepper

For the base

150g (5½oz) ground flaxseeds / linseeds, or any other ground seeds (or see recipe introduction)

70g (2½oz) Cheddar cheese, grated

1 tablespoon olive oil

5 tablespoons water

sea salt flakes

VEGETARIAN

PER SERVING (2 SLICES)	
NET CARBS	10G
FIBRE	14G
PROTEIN	35G
FAT	39G
KCAL	519

A deliciously brilliant way to use up any leftover vegetables, especially at the end of the week when provisions are a little depleted. This is a filling dish and perfect for lunch or dinner. You can select whatever roasted vegetables you prefer, but I suggest sticking to low-starch veg (see page 78 for a list of these), as they are lower in calories and carbohydrates. The ground flaxseed can be replaced with any other ground seed mixes you find in your local supermarket or health food shop, or you can use buckwheat flour, gram flour or any other gluten-free flour instead, but bear in mind that the net carbs will increase.

1 Preheat the oven to 180°C (350°F), Gas Mark 4.

2 If you don't have any leftover roasted vegetables, roast some now (see below).

3 For the base, place the ground seeds, Cheddar, olive oil and a pinch of salt in a mixing bowl and combine together. Add the measured water a little at a time until a dough is formed. (You may not need all 5 tablespoons.)

4 Press the dough into a 22cm (8½ inch) diameter quiche tin or pie dish and prick it with a fork. Place in the oven for 10 minutes to bake, then remove from the oven.

5 Meanwhile, for the filling, place the eggs, coconut milk and a pinch of pepper in a bowl and whisk them together. Pour the mixture into the pastry case and arrange the roasted vegetables and crumbled feta on top.

6 Bake for 20–25 minutes until the filling is firm, then carefully remove from the oven and allow to cool. This quiche will keep in the refrigerator for up to 3 days.

RECIPE TIP
To roast vegetables, preheat the oven to 180°C (350°F), Gas Mark 4. Toss roughly chopped low-starch vegetables (such as red onion, courgette or pepper) with olive oil and salt in a roasting dish, then roast for 35 minutes, turning after 20 minutes.

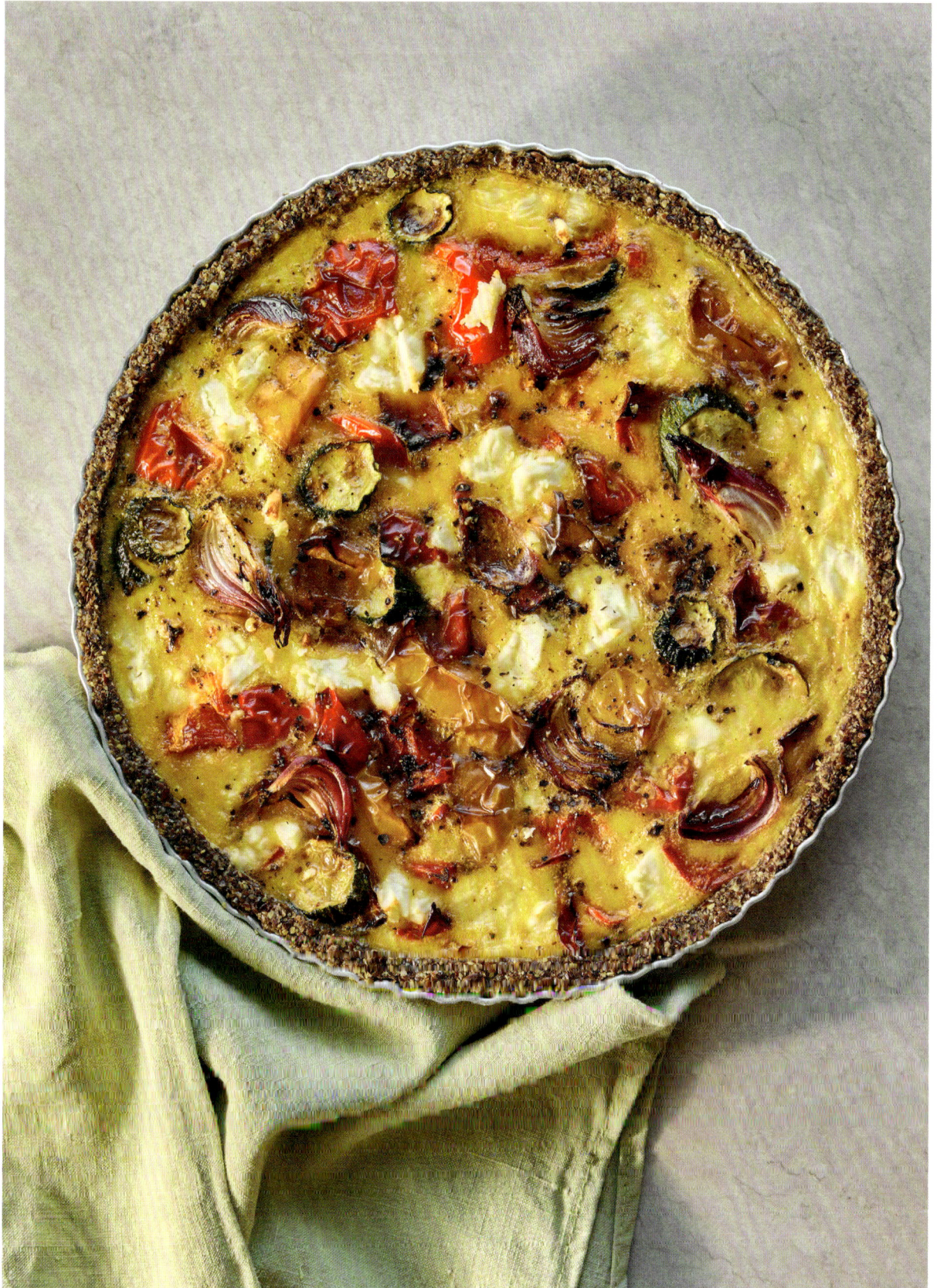

SUMMER PRAWN AND MANGO SALSA BOWL

SERVES
4

PREP TIME
10 MINS

COOK TIME
5 MINS

For the prawns

340g (12oz) raw king prawns, shelled

½ teaspoon garlic purée

½ teaspoon deseeded and finely
   chopped red chilli

2 tablespoons lime juice

1 teaspoon olive oil

For the salsa

1 small mango, peeled and finely
   chopped

1 shallot, finely chopped

1 tablespoon chopped fresh coriander
   leaves, plus more to serve

finely grated zest of 1 lime, plus
   1 tablespoon lime juice

sea salt flakes

To serve

4 handfuls of mixed salad leaves

100g (3½oz) red cabbage, shredded

1 avocado, peeled, pitted and sliced

1 lime, quartered

This is a quick and mouth-watering meal, using only fresh ingredients. Any leftovers are great packed into an airtight container, refrigerated, then taken with you as a packed lunch on the next day.

1 Place the king prawns in a bowl. Add the garlic purée, chilli, lime juice and olive oil. Mix together.

2 Put the mango in a separate bowl with the shallot, coriander, lime zest and juice and a pinch of salt. Mix together.

3 Tip the prawns and their marinade into a frying pan and set over a medium heat. Cook for 2–3 minutes on each side until opaque, pink and cooked through. Set aside.

4 Place a handful of salad leaves on each plate and divide the cabbage and avocado among them. Add the mango salsa and prawns, scattering with a few more coriander leaves and adding a lime quarter. Dig in!

PER SERVING	
NET CARBS	8.6G
FIBRE	3.4G
PROTEIN	17G
FAT	8.3G
KCAL	189

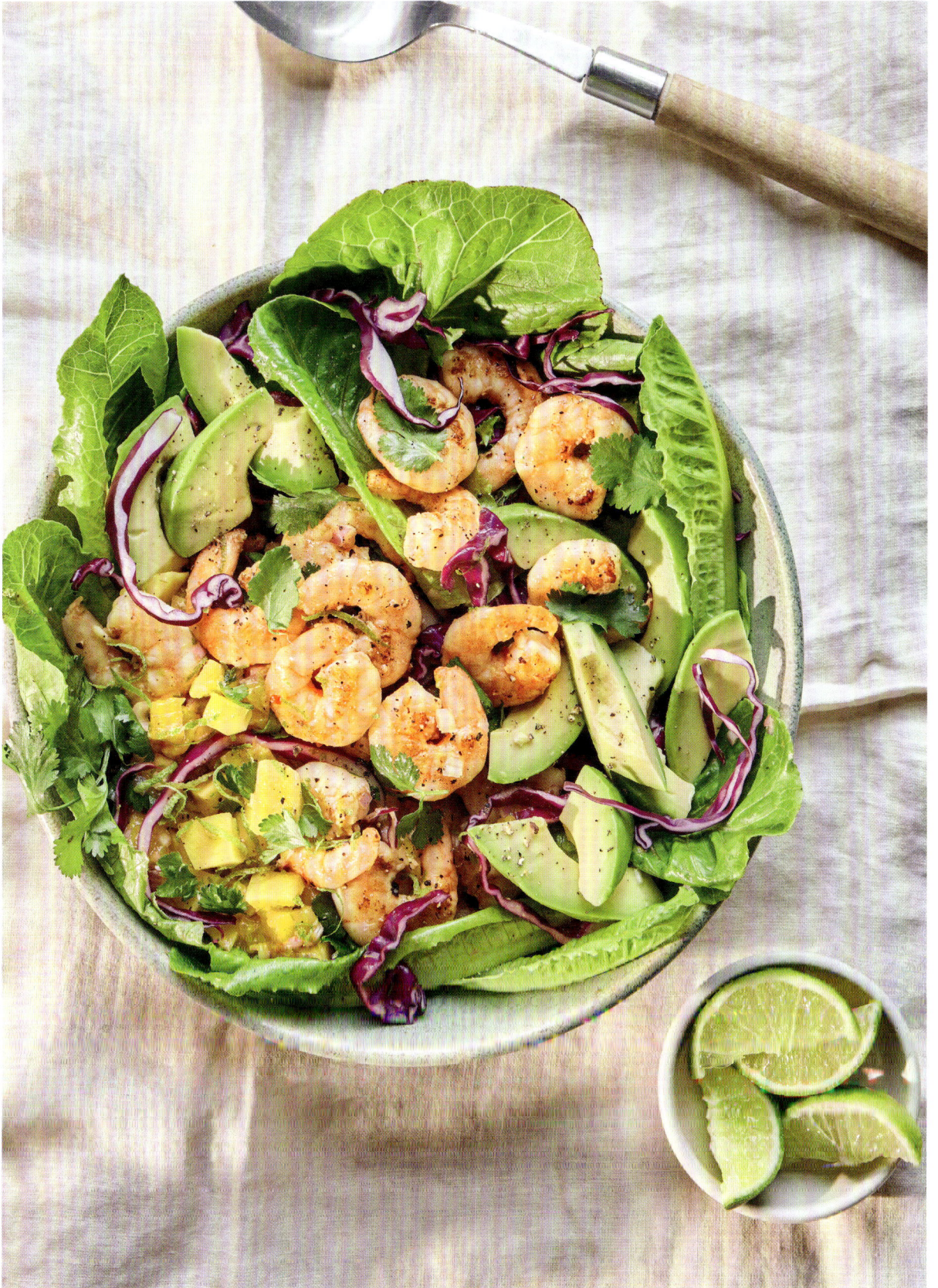

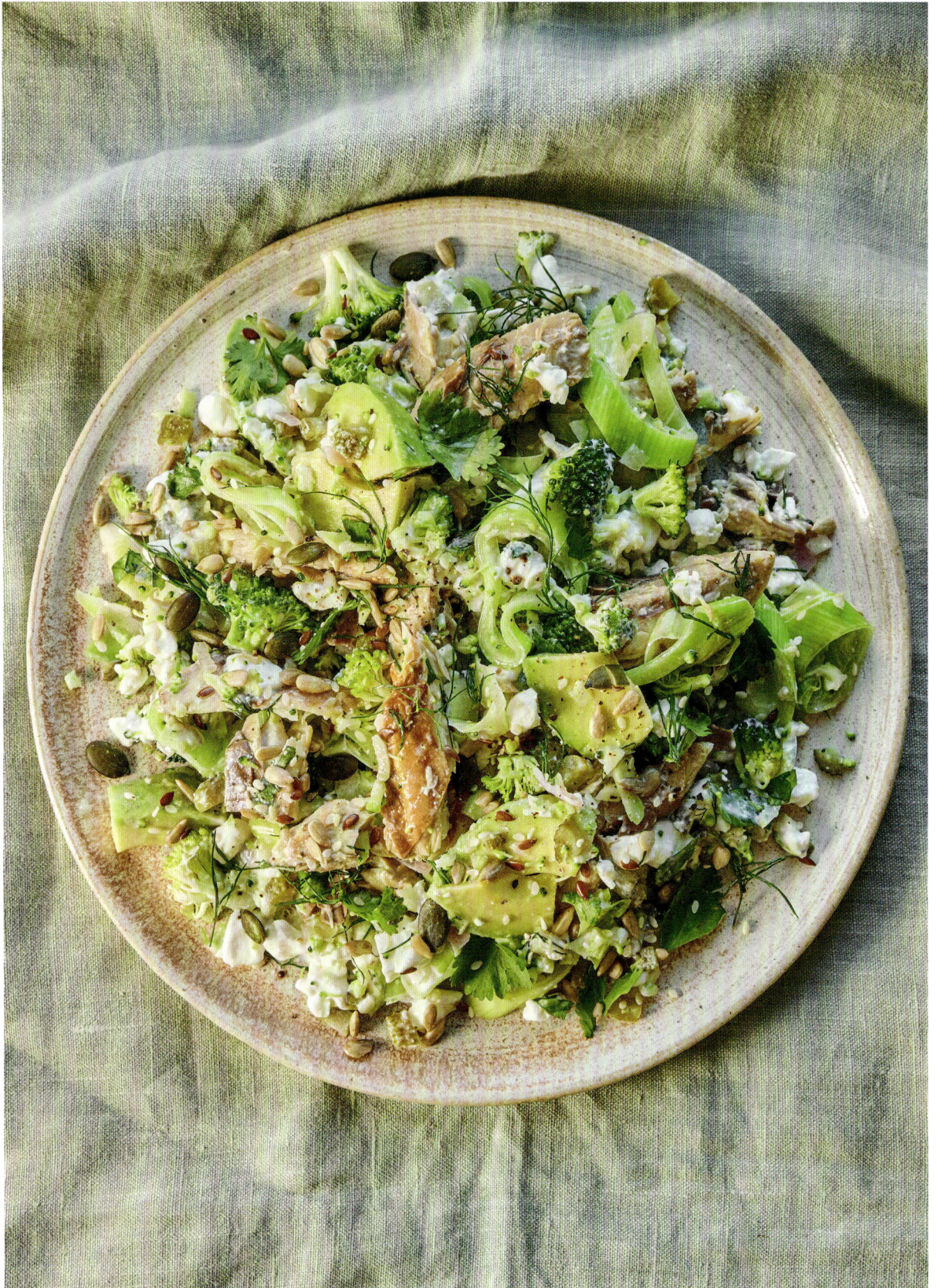

CHOPPED SALAD OF MACKEREL
WITH CRUNCHY GREENS

SERVES
4

PREP TIME
15 MINS

COOK TIME
5 MINS

1 teaspoon light olive oil

1 teaspoon unsalted butter

130g (4½oz) leeks, finely sliced

60g (2¼oz) shallots, finely chopped

120g (4¼oz) broccoli

1 tablespoon chopped dill

1 tablespoon chopped fresh coriander leaves

30g (1oz) avocado, chopped

110g (3¾oz) pickled gherkins, chopped

10g (¼oz) mixed seeds

110g (3¾oz) cottage cheese

80g (2¾oz) mackerel in water or brine, drained

2 tablespoons apple cider vinegar

sea salt flakes

Chopped salads are very popular and this recipe has a blend of raw and cooked flavoursome ingredients for a perfect crunch. The mackerel and cottage cheese provide protein. If you would prefer this salad to be vegan, omit the mackerel and add some roasted butternut squash or sweet potato. Alternatively, another oily fish such as sardines would work, or a cheese such as feta or halloumi instead of cottage cheese.

1 Heat the oil and butter in a frying pan, add the leeks and shallots and cook until soft, translucent and fragrant (about 5 minutes). Set aside.

2 Finely chop the broccoli on a chopping board to a rice-like consistency. Pop it into a mixing bowl and add the dill, coriander, avocado and gherkins. Stir in the cooled leeks and shallots.

3 Add a generous pinch of sea salt, the mixed seeds, cottage cheese, mackerel and vinegar. Mix together well until combined.

4 Serve straight away, or put in an airtight container for another time and eat within 24 hours.

NET CARBS	5G
FIBRE	3.3G
PROTEIN	9.5G
FAT	11G
KCAL	163

FISH AND SEAFOOD

SUSHI ROLLS, 2 WAYS

SERVES
4

PREP TIME
20 MINS

COOK TIME
7 MINS

For the rice

300g (10½oz) cauliflower

olive oil spray

60g (2¼oz) cream cheese

1 teaspoon apple cider vinegar

For the spicy tuna filling

2 x 145g (5¼oz) cans of tuna in water, drained

2 tablespoons mayonnaise

1 teaspoon sriracha

1 teaspoon apple cider vinegar

1 teaspoon chilli flakes

1 teaspoon chilli oil (optional)

For the salmon filling

70g (2½oz) smoked salmon, sliced, or sliced salmon sashimi

½ cucumber, sliced

½ avocado, sliced

To serve

2–3 sheets of nori seaweed

1 teaspoon black sesame seeds

root ginger or pickled sushi ginger

low-salt soy sauce

PER SERVING	TUNA	SALMON
NET CARBS	9.6G	10G
FIBRE	1.7G	2.8G
PROTEIN	17G	8.5G
FAT	15G	12G
KCAL	238	183

A simple low-calorie lunch. I adore sushi, but unfortunately rice spikes my blood sugars to the point where all the enjoyment of the meal is lost. However, I've spent lots of time experimenting with alternative ingredients and I'm delighted to tell you that cauliflower 'rice', cooked as shown below, will have the same bite and structure as regular rice. It holds together beautifully, so you can dip the rolls into soy sauce as you would with traditional sushi. Ideally, make the cauliflower 'rice' in advance, so it has chilled by the time you are ready to roll and eat the sushi.

1 Break the cauliflower into florets and place in a food processor. Pulse-blend into a coarse rice-like consistency. Or grate the cauliflower using a box grater (mind your knuckles!).

2 Place a large nonstick frying pan over a medium-high heat and add a spray of olive oil and the cauliflower 'rice'. Cook for about 7 minutes until the cauliflower is tender.

3 Place the warm cauliflower in a bowl with the cream cheese and vinegar. Mix well and refrigerate to cool completely (around 30 minutes).

4 For the spicy tuna filling, place all the ingredients in a small bowl and mix well.

5 Place a nori sheet on a bamboo sushi mat or a clean tea cloth, shiny-side down, and top with some of the cooled cauliflower rice mix. Spread the rice evenly on to the sheet, leaving a 2–3cm (¾–1¼ inch) gap along one long side.

6 Add your chosen filling ingredients in a line lengthways across the centre of the rectangle of rice and roll firmly, until you reach the edge of the rice and the clear nori border. Rub a wet finger on the border and continue to roll firmly to seal it up, pressing through the mat or tea towel as much as you can. Place in the fridge until required. Repeat to roll all the rice and sushi.

7 Cut each roll into about 8 slices. Serve topped with black sesame seeds, with a side of pickled ginger and soy sauce.

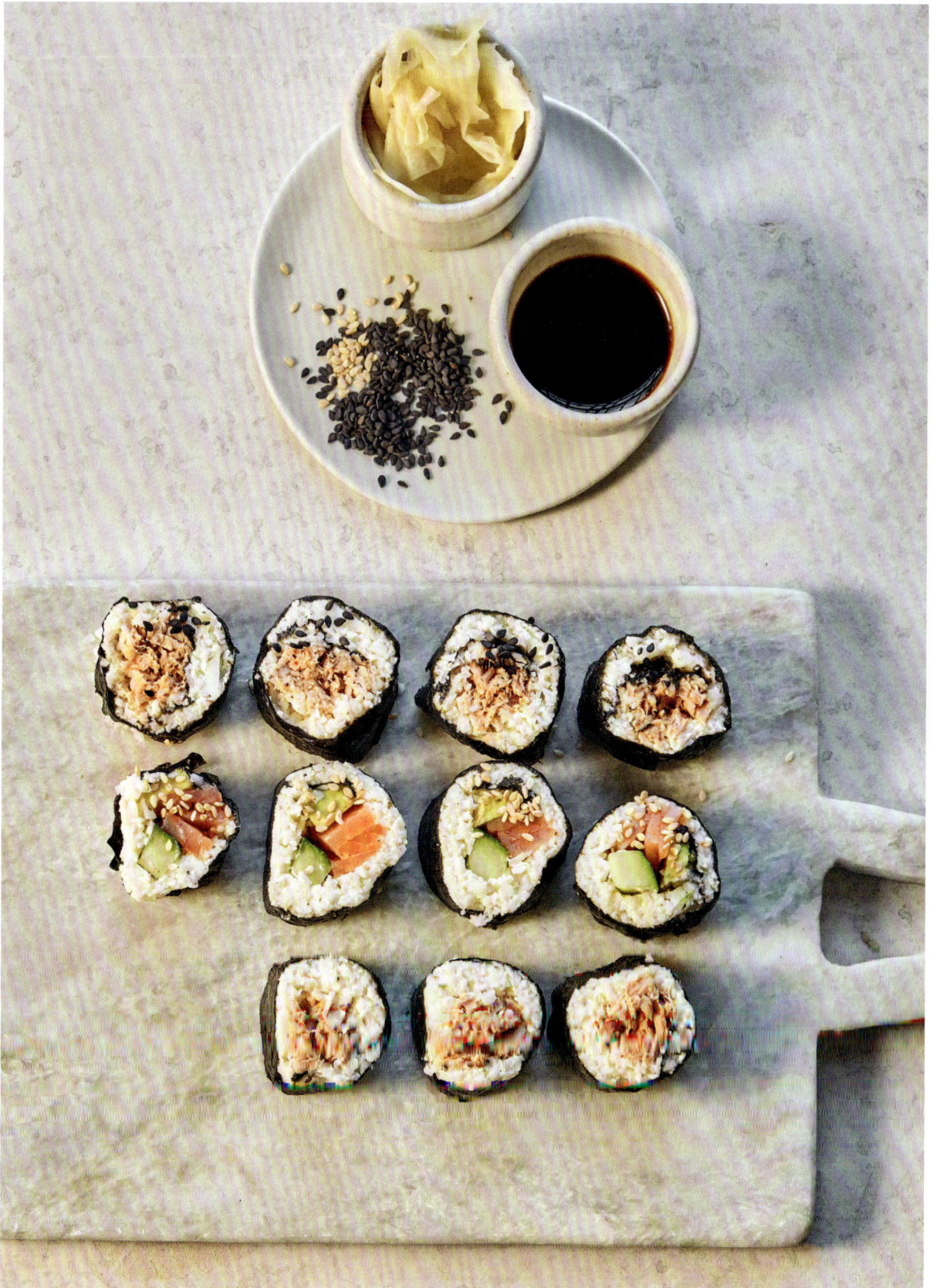

BAKED LEMON AND GARLIC SALMON PARCEL

SERVES
2

1 tablespoon olive oil

2 salmon fillets

1 lemon

2 garlic cloves, finely grated or
   finely chopped

½ teaspoon sea salt flakes

½ teaspoon freshly ground
   black pepper

PER SERVING	
NET CARBS	1G
FIBRE	0.5G
PROTEIN	24G
FAT	19G
KCAL	277

PREP TIME
5 MINS

COOK TIME
20 MINS

One of the quickest and most simple ways to cook and enjoy a salmon fillet. This is a nutritious meal and works perfectly with Cauliflower 'couscous' (see page 12) a handful of salad leaves (such as rocket) or stir-fried greens. Prepping ahead is always a good idea, and by cooking two fillets at a time you can enjoy one for dinner and pop the other in the refrigerator, still sealed in the foil, to eat for lunch the next day with a mixed leaf salad.

1 Preheat the oven to 180°C (350°F), Gas Mark 4.

2 Pour the oil on to a piece of foil large enough to parcel up the salmon. Rub the salmon fillets in the oil on both sides, then place them on the foil with the skin side underneath.

3 Roll the lemon firmly under the heel of your hand (this makes it easier to juice), then cut it in half and squeeze about 1 tablespoon juice over each salmon fillet. Slice up the rest of the lemon. Rub half the garlic over each fillet, add a generous pinch of salt and a pinch of black pepper and place the lemon slices on top.

4 Seal up the foil into a parcel and bake for 20 minutes.

5 Remove from the oven, checking the centre has cooked through, and serve immediately, or allow to cool and place it into the refrigerator, still sealed in its foil, and eat within 24 hours.

RECIPE TIP

I like to serve the baked lemon slices with my salmon, as the lemon soaks up a lot of the flavour and is delicious. Alternatively, serve this with some fresh lemon slices.

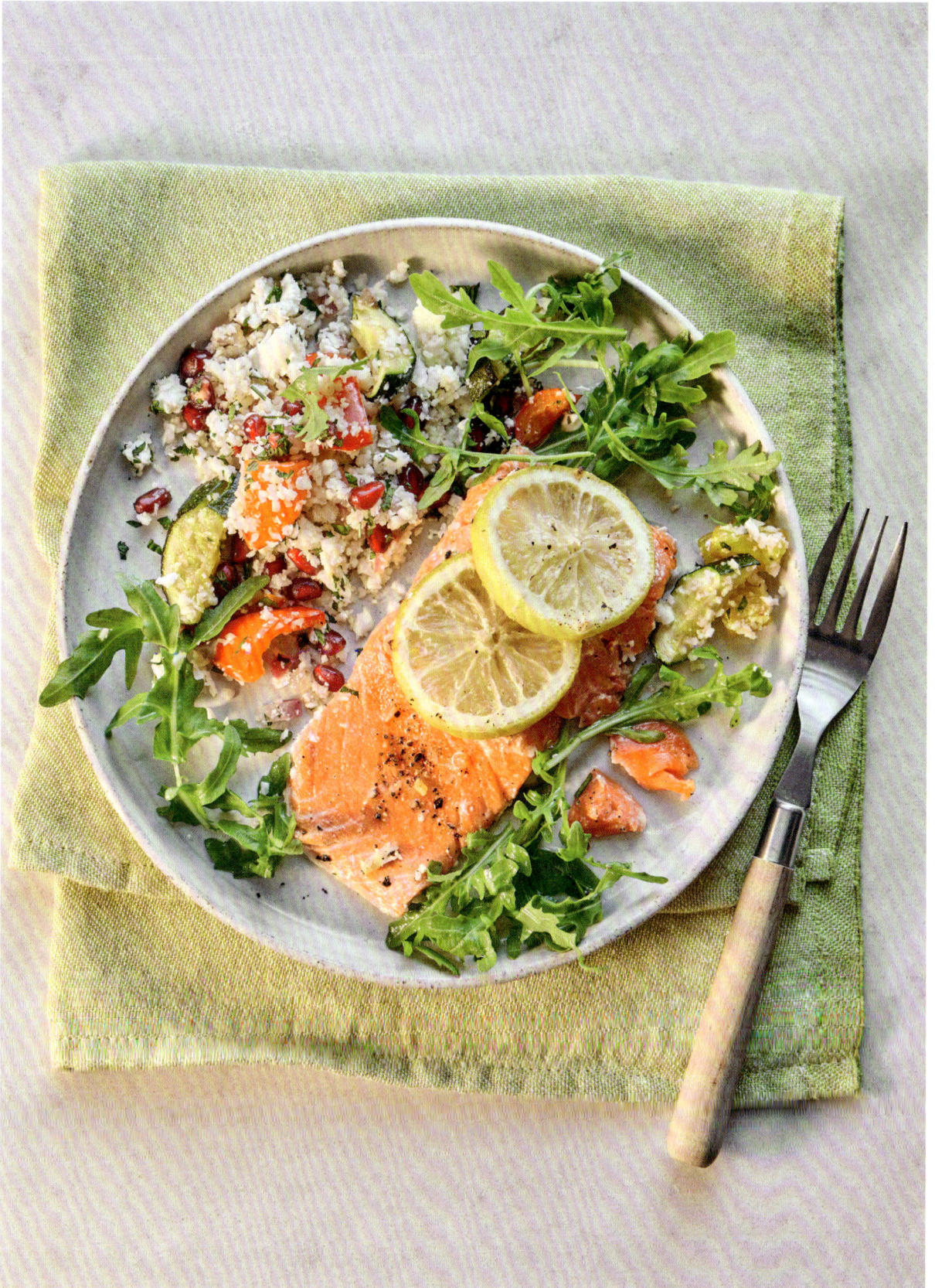

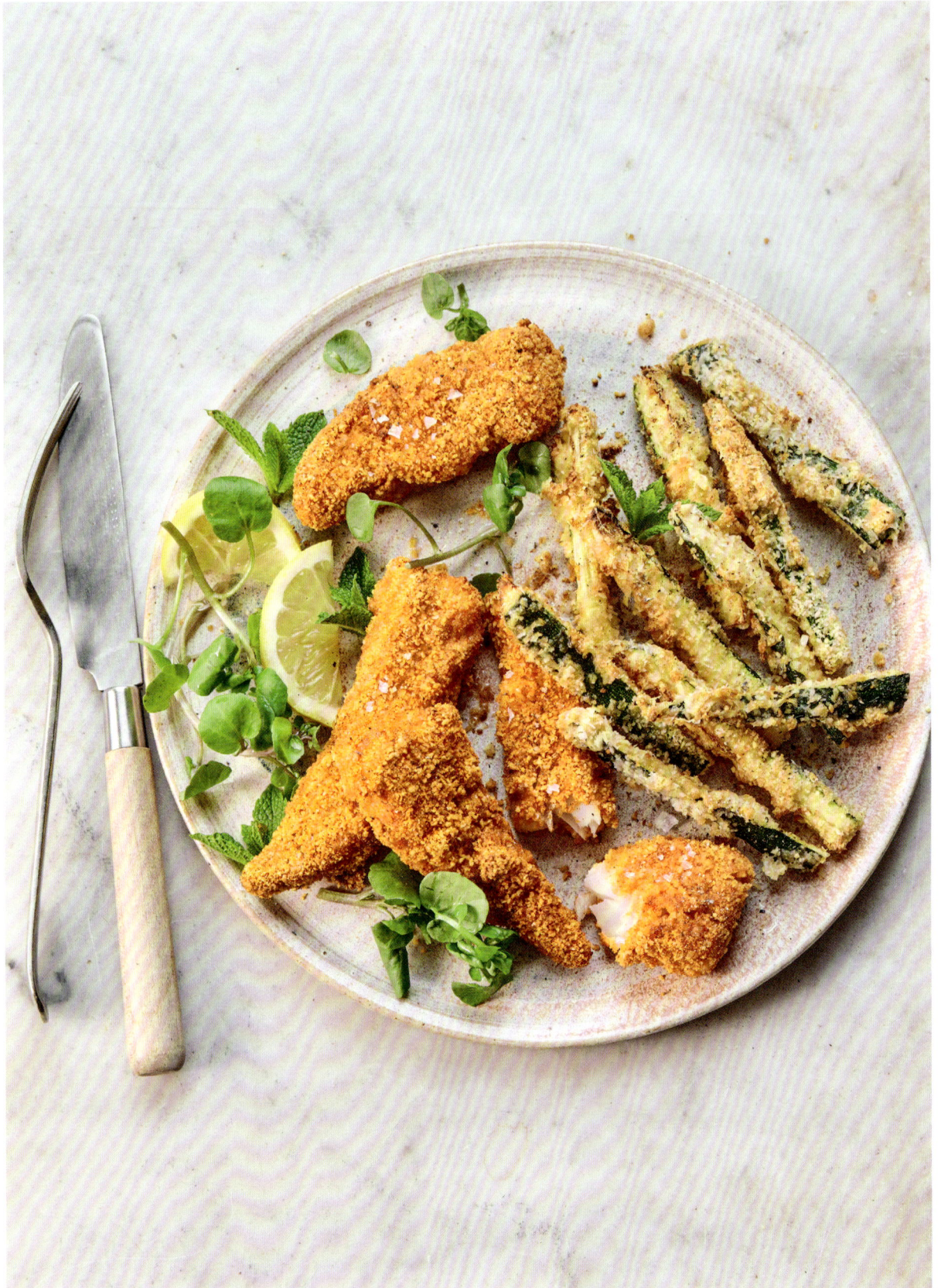

CRISPY FISH GOUJONS

SERVES
2

PREP TIME
15 MINS

COOK TIME
15 MINS

1 large egg

40g (1½oz) ground almonds

2 teaspoons paprika

1 teaspoon onion powder

2 pinches of sea salt flakes

pinch of freshly ground black pepper

300g (10½oz) cod fillets, or any other white fish fillets, cut into goujons

1 teaspoon coconut oil

PER SERVING	
NET CARBS	2.5G
FIBRE	2.9G
PROTEIN	35G
FAT	17G
KCAL	308

For some reason, in the UK, 6pm in the evening is the most likely time that supermarkets discount fish. Just give it a go at that time and you can often pick up a few packs of heavily discounted white fish fillets and pop them straight into the freezer for a rainy day. Whether its cod, haddock or hake, they all work well in this recipe. Fish fingers are a quick and easy supper for children, and when you make them yourself they are more nutritious than shop-bought. Adults, of course, love them, too. You can make these with chicken or turkey if you prefer. Serve with Smoky Sweet Potato Fries (see page 124), to create a healthier twist on fish fingers or chicken nuggets and chips.

1 Preheat the oven to 180°C (350°F), Gas Mark 4 and line a baking sheet with nonstick baking paper.

2 Break the egg into a shallow bowl and lightly beat it. Place the ground almonds, paprika, onion powder, sea salt and pepper on a separate dinner plate. Mix these together until well combined.

3 Chop the fish into goujons. Take a goujon, dip it into the egg, then roll it in the paprika mix. Repeat to coat all the goujons.

4 Put the coconut oil into a frying pan over a medium heat and allow it to melt. Once melted, add the goujons. Allow one side to cook for 2 minutes before flipping them over and cooking the other side.

5 Once they are a golden brown colour, place them on a baking sheet and finish off in the oven for 5–8 minutes until fully cooked. (Check a thicker goujon to make sure the centre is piping hot and the fish is thoroughly cooked.) Serve immediately.

PAD THAI WITH KING PRAWNS

SERVES
2

PREP TIME
10 MINS

COOK TIME
10 MINS

3 tablespoons fish sauce

2 tablespoons sweetener

1 tablespoon lime juice

1 tablespoon tamari sauce

1 tablespoon apple cider vinegar

200g (7oz) konjac noodles (see below and recipe introduction)

1 tablespoon sesame oil

150g (5½oz) beansprouts

200g (7oz) cooked king prawns

2 garlic cloves, crushed

150g (5½oz) pak choi

To serve

handful of fresh coriander leaves

20g (¾oz) peanuts, chopped and toasted

2 spring onions, finely sliced

1 lime, cut into wedges

PER SERVING	
NET CARBS	9G
FIBRE	4.2G
PROTEIN	25G
FAT	13G
KCAL	267

The perfect fakeaway: a healthier takeaway! If you do not want to use shirataki noodles (see below), try courgette 'noodles' (see page 58), added at the end just to flash-fry into the pad Thai ingredients (don't overcook them, or they will become too soft). You could also try shredded white cabbage ribbons, added at the same time as you would add the shirataki noodles and allowed to soften for a couple of minutes before serving, or even cauliflower 'rice' (see page 84).

1 Mix the fish sauce, sweetener, lime juice, tamari and vinegar in a small bowl.

2 Prepare the shirataki noodles according to the instructions on the packet. Set aside.

3 Place the sesame oil into a wok over a medium-high heat. Add the beansprouts and soften. Once softened, toss in the prawns and garlic and cook for 2 minutes. Throw in the pak choi and allow to wilt. Once wilted, add the sauce from the small bowl and bring to a bubble for a couple of minutes.

4 Once the sauce has started to thicken, add the shirataki noodles and flash-fry in the sauce for a few minutes.

5 Serve immediately with coriander, scattered with peanuts and spring onions and a lime wedge.

RECIPE TIP

Konjac noodles are also known as shirataki noodles or 'skinny noodles'. They are made from the corm of the konjac plant and are available in most major supermarkets, health food shops and Asian markets. These are brilliant for those living with diabetes, as they are not only 0 carb but they also contain only 10 calories per serving, so are the perfect dish for weight management. They are also high in fibre, which means they keep you full.

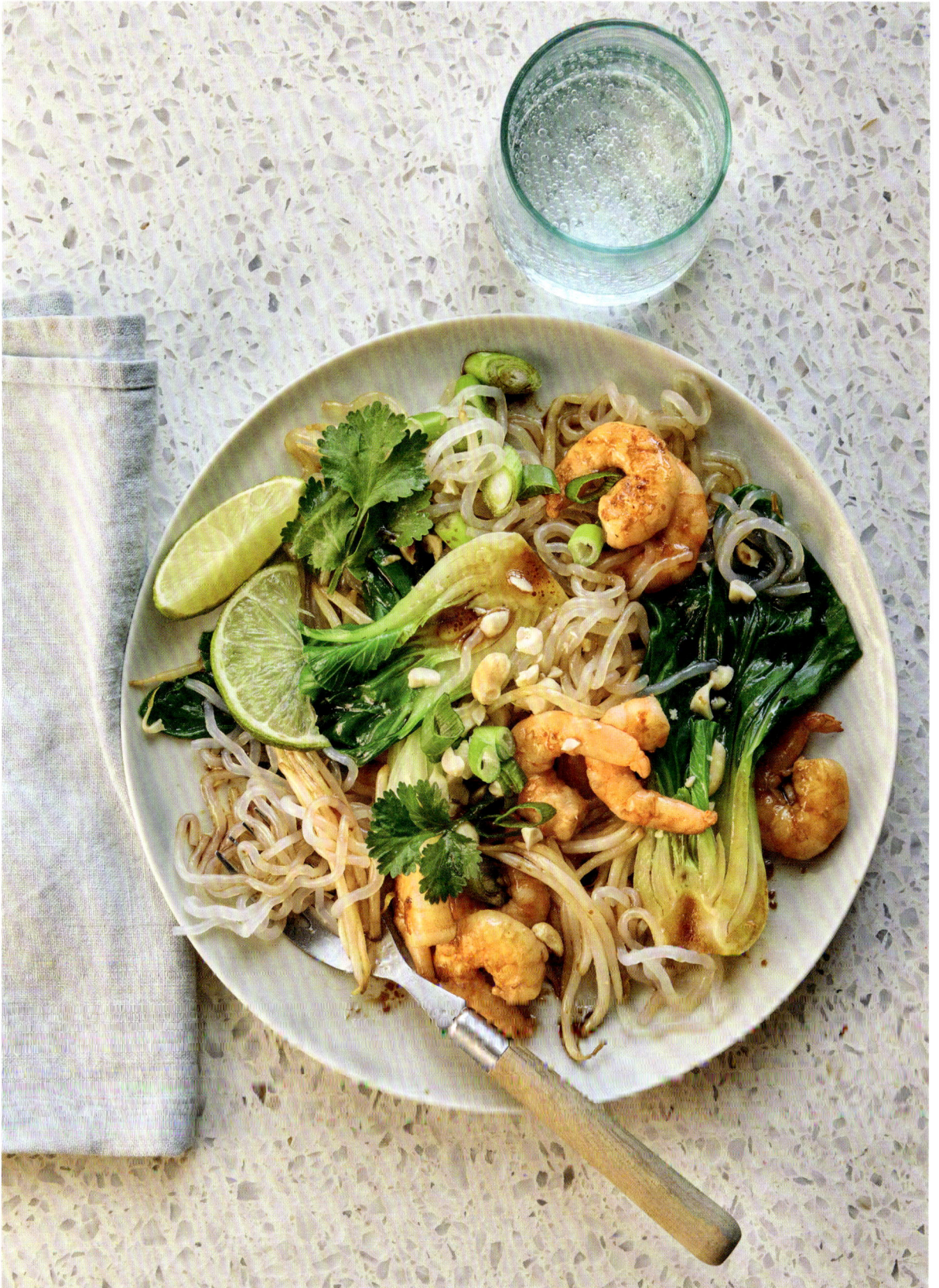

FISH PIE WITH A CELERIAC AND BROCCOLI TOPPING

SERVES
6

PREP TIME
20 MINS

COOK TIME
1 HOUR

For the topping

250g (9oz) celeriac, peeled and cut into rough chunks

400g (14oz) broccoli, cut into florets, tough stalks removed

3 tablespoons unsalted butter

handful of flat leaf parsley leaves, chopped

3 tablespoons grated Parmesan cheese

sea salt flakes and cracked black pepper

For the filling

25g (1oz) unsalted butter

2 spring onions (total weight about 30g / 1oz), roughly chopped

100g (3½oz) leeks, sliced

20g (¾oz) celery sticks, finely chopped

25g (1oz) coconut flour or arrowroot or gluten-free plain flour

400ml (14fl oz) can of coconut milk

50g (1¾oz) Cheddar cheese, grated

420g (15oz) mixture of boneless fish pie mix (I use a mix of cod, smoked haddock and salmon) and prawns

100g (3½oz) frozen or fresh peas

PER SERVING	
NET CARBS	9.4G
FIBRE	8G
PROTEIN	25G
FAT	31G
KCAL	430

The ultimate comfort food. This ticks every box, as it is full of flavour and jam-packed with protein, healthy fats and lots of fibre, but also low in carbs. It can be prepared in advance and chilled for a couple of days or frozen.

1 Preheat the oven to 220°C (425°F), Gas Mark 7.

2 Start by making the topping. Place the celeriac in a saucepan and cover with water. Bring to the boil and simmer for 10 minutes, then add the broccoli and cook for a further 10 minutes until tender. Drain well, then mash with the butter, adding some seasoning and three-quarters of the chopped parsley. Set aside.

3 Now, start on the filling. Place the butter, spring onions, leeks and celery in a deep-sided saucepan set over a low heat, cover and sweat (cook without colouring) for 3–4 minutes until softened. Stir in the coconut flour using a wooden spoon, then gradually add the coconut milk and whisk until fully incorporated and there are no lumps left in the mixture. Increase the heat and cook until the mixture has reached boiling point, then reduce the heat and cook at a gentle simmer for 3–4 minutes until thickened.

4 Remove the pan from the heat and stir in the Cheddar, fish and peas and season with salt and pepper. Pour the fish mixture into a baking dish and spoon the broccoli mash on top, using a fork to level it out.

5 Place into the oven and cook for 20 minutes. Preheat the grill.

6 After 20 minutes, carefully remove the pie from the oven, scatter over the Parmesan and remaining parsley, then place it under the hot grill to crisp the surface for a maximum of 10 minutes.

7 Once bubbling and golden, allow to rest for 5 minutes before serving. Or allow it to fully cool, cover, then chill. The pie will keep in the refrigerator for 2–3 days, or you can freeze it.

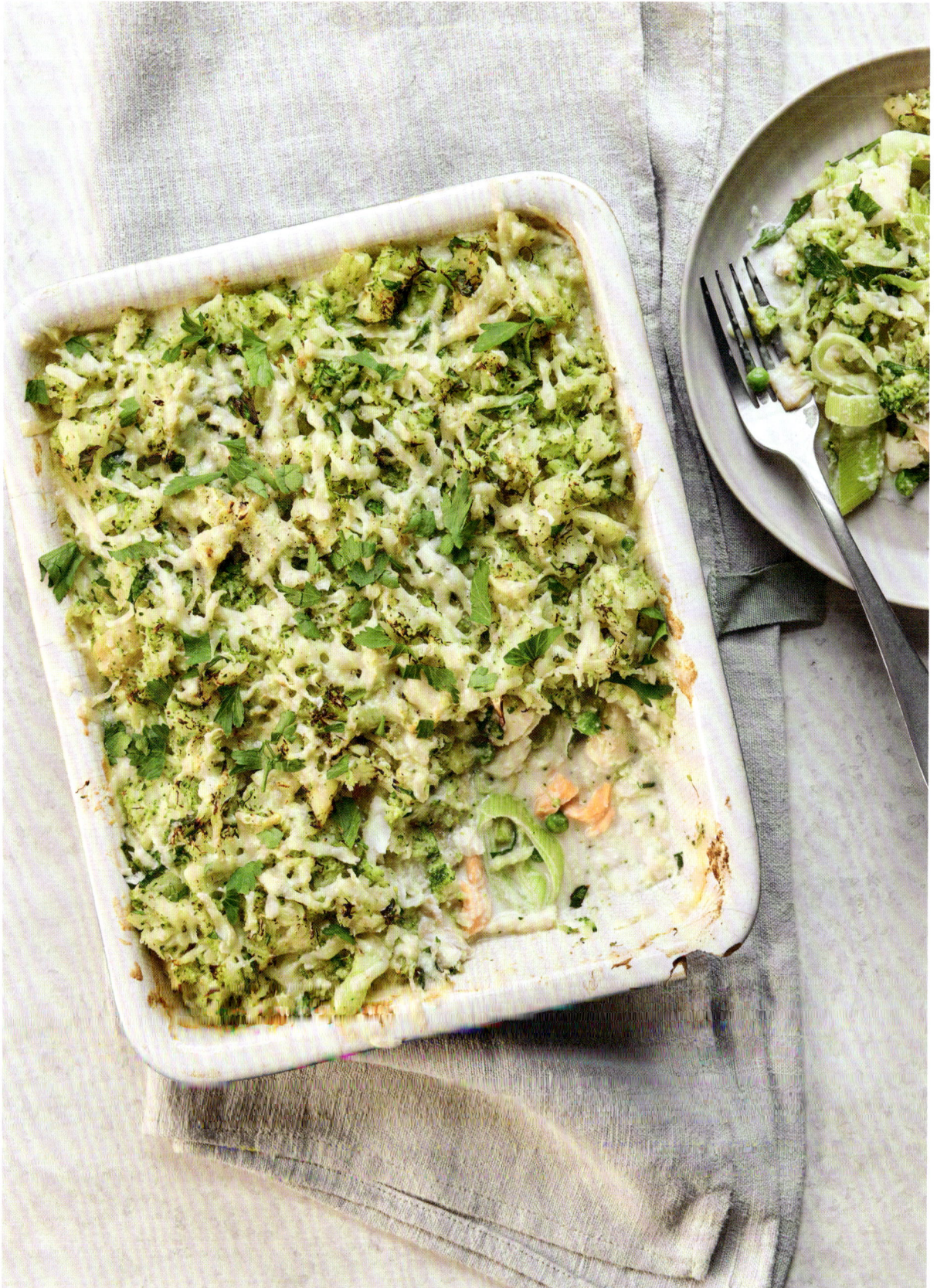

PERFECT STEAK WITH MUSHROOM PEPPER SAUCE AND A SIMPLE SALAD

SERVES	**PREP TIME**	**COOK TIME**
2	15 MINS	15 MINS

For the steaks

2 x 280g (10oz) grass-fed sirloin steaks at room temperature (or see below)

2 tablespoons light olive oil

2 teaspoons sea salt flakes

2 teaspoons cracked black pepper

For the salad

100g (3½oz) mixed salad leaves

1 spring onion, chopped

70g (2½oz) cucumber, sliced

olive oil spray

1 tablespoon apple cider vinegar

1 tablespoon balsamic vinegar

For the sauce

30g (1oz) unsalted butter

130g (4½oz) chestnut mushrooms, finely sliced

2 small shallots, finely chopped

1 teaspoon very finely chopped or finely grated garlic

1 teaspoon cracked black pepper

2 tablespoons water

2 tablespoons soured cream

PER SERVING	
NET CARBS	6G
FIBRE	2.7G
PROTEIN	70G
FAT	44G
KCAL	706

Simple food is often the best and this is absolute perfection. This is a testament to my husband: he grew up in pubs and his mum was a chef, so he is truly magnificent at not only being the quickest and most efficient washer-upper, but he also is brilliant at making typical pub grub. We both adore steak and so, when the opportunity allows, this is our favourite meal to enjoy together. If you need some chips to go with it, try my Peppery Parmesan Courgette Fries, Roasted Celeriac and Rosemary Roasties or Smoky Sweet Potato Fries (see pages 114, 169 and 124).

1 Place the steaks on a plate and cover with the olive oil. Season with salt and pepper.

2 Place the salad leaves, spring onion and cucumber in a bowl. Spray with olive oil and add the apple cider and balsamic vinegars. Toss together and set aside.

3 Place a nonstick frying pan over a high heat until very hot but not smoking. Add the steaks to the pan and cook for 3 minutes on each side for medium-rare. Finish off the steaks by searing the fatty edges for 1 minute. The fat will melt and add flavour. Set aside on a plate and leave to rest for around 5 minutes while you make the mushroom sauce.

4 In the same pan over a medium heat, melt the butter and soften the mushrooms and shallots for 2 minutes. Add the garlic and pepper and cook for a further minute, adding the juices from the rested steaks. Add the measured water to deglaze the pan, then after 30 seconds remove from the heat and stir in the soured cream until you have a light brown, creamy sauce.

5 Place a generous handful of salad on to warmed plates and add the steaks. Spoon the mushroom sauce over the steaks and serve.

RECIPE TIP You can use any cut of steak, just be mindful that each cut will need a different cooking time.

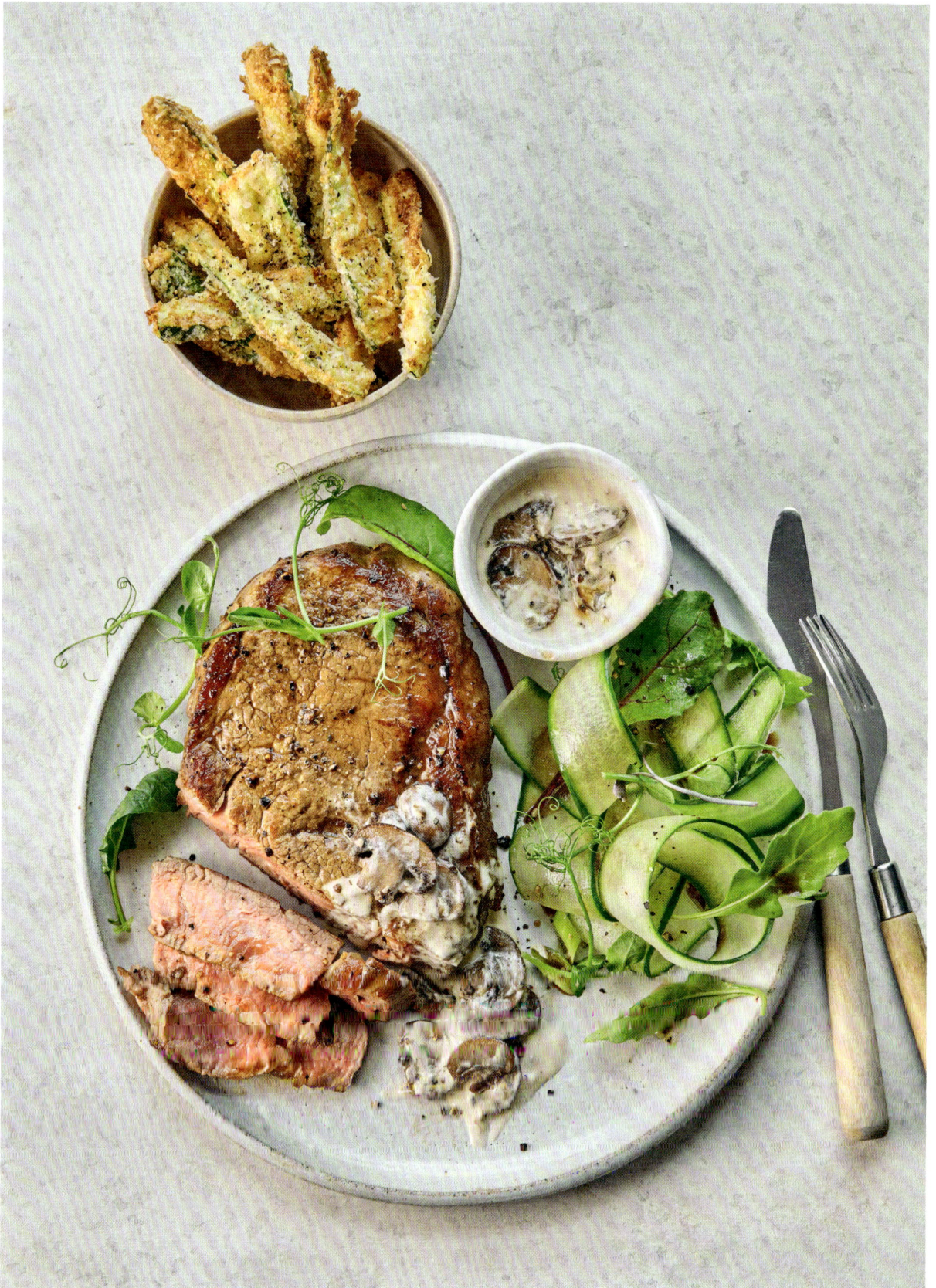

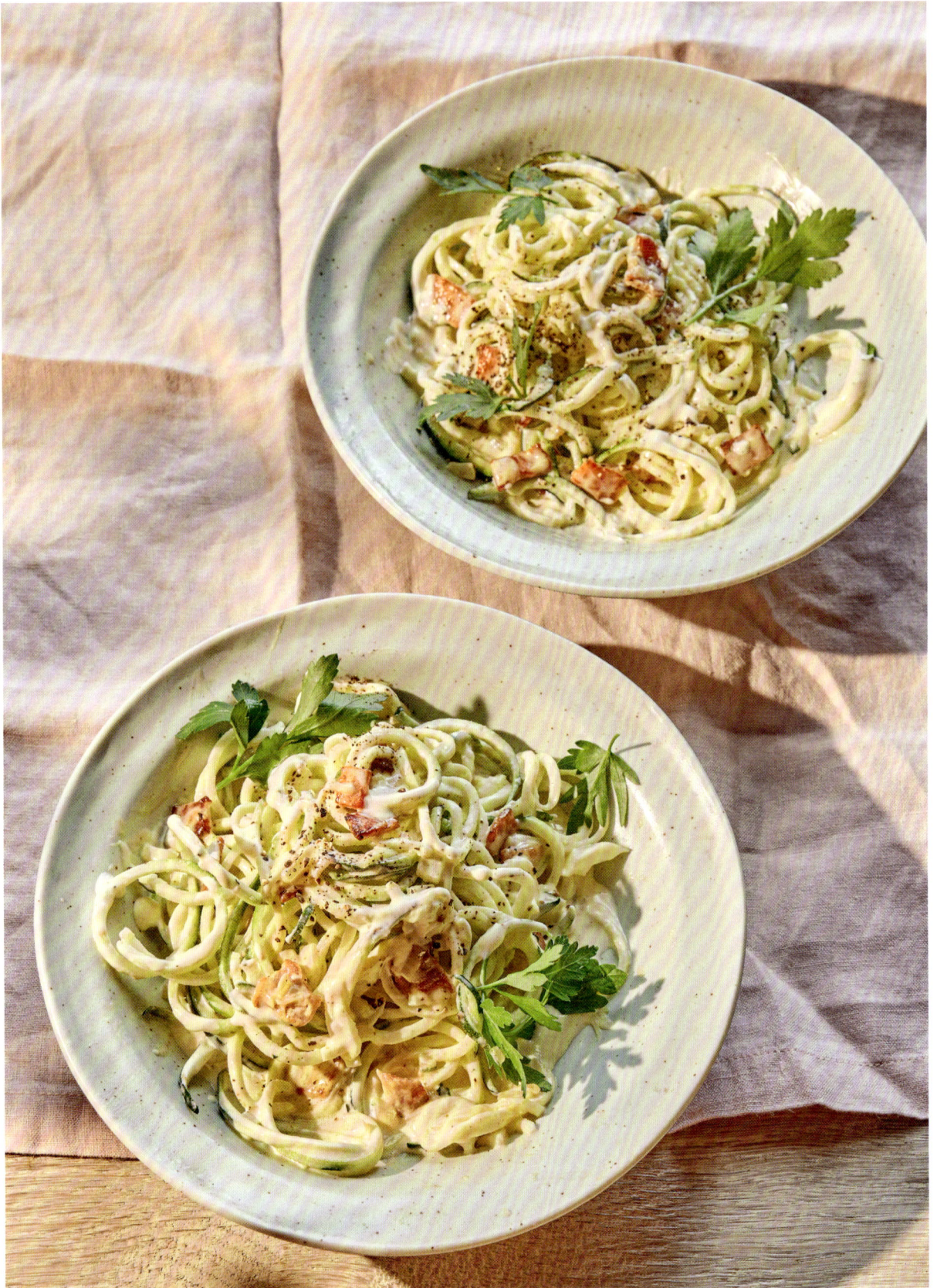

CREAMY COURGETTE CARBONARA

SERVES
2

PREP TIME
10 MINS

COOK TIME
10 MINS

1 tablespoon unsalted butter

1 onion, finely chopped

1 spring onion, sliced

50g (1¾oz) bacon, trimmed of fat, chopped

200ml (7fl oz) low-fat coconut milk

30g (1oz) mature grated Cheddar cheese

pinch of cracked black pepper

2 large courgettes, spiralized into 'noodles' (see page 58 and the recipe introduction)

handful of flat leaf parsley leaves, to serve (optional)

Here, I've focused on creating a creamy, appetizing, filling and nutritionally dense meal, but have kept the carb content as low as possible by using simple, wholesome ingredients. This recipe contains all the delights of eating noodles, without the high blood sugars. If you are not keen on courgettes, you can replace them with a low-carb alternative such as shirataki noodles (see page 142), or even use a smaller portion (50g / 1¾oz) of wholewheat noodles instead. Use a low-fat cheese, if you need to.

1 Place the butter in a deep frying pan and melt over a medium-high heat. Fry the onion, spring onion and bacon until soft.

2 Reduce the heat, add the coconut milk and cheese and stir through. Cook for a few minutes until the mix has thickened slightly.

3 Add the black pepper and courgette noodles and stir again.

4 Scatter with parsley, if you like, then serve.

PER SERVING	
NET CARBS	11G
FIBRE	2.6G
PROTEIN	15G
FAT	27G
KCAL	353

MEAT

THAI TURKEY BURGERS, CRUNCHY SLAW AND SRIRACHA SAUCE

SERVES
4

PREP TIME
30 MINS, PLUS CHILLING
AND RESTING TIME

COOK TIME
15 MINS

For the burgers

400g (14oz) lean minced turkey

½ lemongrass stalk, finely chopped

1 shallot, finely chopped

1 garlic clove, crushed

2.5cm (1 inch) fresh root ginger, grated

1 red chilli, finely chopped

finely grated zest and juice of ½ lime

5g (¼oz) fresh coriander, chopped,
   plus more to serve

olive oil

sea salt flakes and black pepper

For the slaw

80g (2¾oz) red cabbage, shredded

80g (2¾oz) cucumber ribbons (see
   page 118)

80g (2¾oz) carrot, grated

2 spring onions, finely sliced

finely grated zest and juice of 1 lime

1 teaspoon Dijon mustard

olive oil spray

For the sriracha sauce

80g (2¾oz) Greek yogurt

1 tablespoon sriracha

A real crowd-pleaser, bursting with Thai flavours. If you are having a feast with your family or friends, you could add some Smoky Sweet Potato Fries (see page 124), leaving out the paprika and replacing the olive oil with sesame oil, to provide extra colour and heartiness. Burger buns tend to be highly processed, full of salt and additives and high in carbs, which can spike blood sugars. You might prefer to use large firm lettuce leaves, such as Romaine, as a wrap for the burgers, if needed.

1 Combine all the ingredients for the burgers except the oil in a bowl with a generous pinch of salt and mix together well. With wet hands, shape the ingredients into 4 burgers. Place on a plate and refrigerate for 20 minutes.

2 Preheat the oven to 180°C (350°F), Gas Mark 4. Oil a baking tray.

3 Put a little olive oil in a griddle pan or frying pan over a medium heat. Add the burgers to the pan and cook for about 4 minutes until golden brown underneath. Flip over and cook the other side until golden brown. Transfer to the prepared baking tray and place in the oven to finish off for about 5 minutes. Set aside to rest for a few minutes before serving.

4 Put all the ingredients for the slaw in a bowl with a couple of sprays of olive oil and toss together.

5 Mix all the ingredients for the sauce in a bowl.

6 Serve the burgers with the slaw and sauce.

PER SERVING	
NET CARBS	6G
FIBRE	2G
PROTEIN	25G
FAT	9.6G
KCAL	216

RECIPE TIP

Cabbage is a brilliant standby vegetable, as it stays fresh in the fridge for up to 3 weeks and is very versatile. You can eat it raw or enjoy it cooked. It makes a great addition to salads, adding crunch, texture and colour, and is brilliant to ferment for sauerkraut.

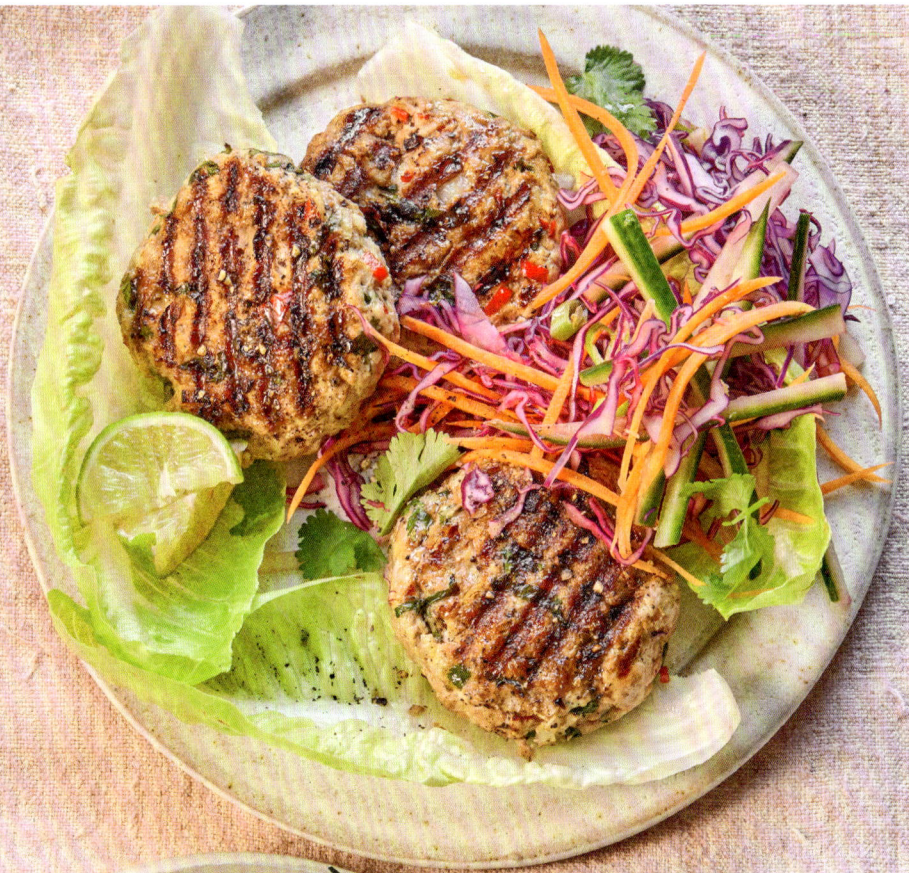

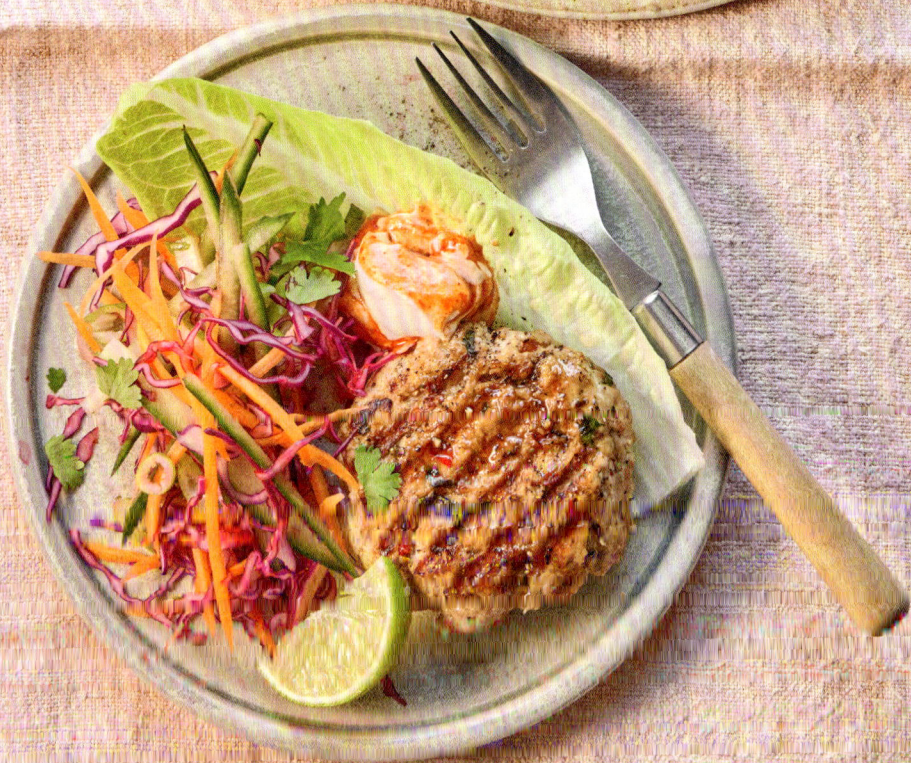

LAMB KOFTAS
WITH MINTED YOGURT DIP

SERVES
4 / MAKES 8

PREP TIME
30 MINS, PLUS MARINATING AND RESTING TIME

COOK TIME
15 MINS

For the koftas

400g (14oz) minced lamb

2 tablespoons harissa paste

50g (1¾oz) sundried tomatoes in oil, chopped

sea salt flakes and freshly ground black pepper

For the dip

100g (3½oz) fat-free additive-free natural yogurt

2 teaspoons finely chopped mint leaves

2 tablespoons lime juice

An absolute winner, popular with the whole family. These koftas are seasoned with harissa paste and combined with sundried tomatoes. Koftas are one of the quickest and easiest recipes to make and a great dish to prepare in advance for the next day. The smell of them cooking will make your mouth water! The dip is fresh, light and creamy.

1 Place 8 wooden skewers into a bowl of cold water to soak for about 20 minutes.

2 Place the lamb, harissa paste, sundried tomatoes, salt and pepper in a bowl and use your hands to combine all the ingredients together.

3 Once combined, take golf ball-sized balls and roll into kofta (sausage-like) shapes. Slide each on to a wooden skewer and arrange on a baking sheet. Set aside for at least 30 minutes to allow the flavours to infuse.

4 Meanwhile, place the yogurt, chopped mint and lime juice in a bowl and mix together. Leave the flavours to infuse.

5 Preheat the oven to 190°C (375°F), Gas Mark 5.

6 Place the koftas into the oven for 8 minutes, then flip them over and cook for a further 5–6 minutes until cooked through. Check regularly and do not overcook. Remove from the oven and rest for a further 5 minutes before serving with the dip.

PER SERVING (2 KOFTAS)	
NET CARBS	3G
FIBRE	1.1G
PROTEIN	23G
FAT	16G
KCAL	249

MEAT

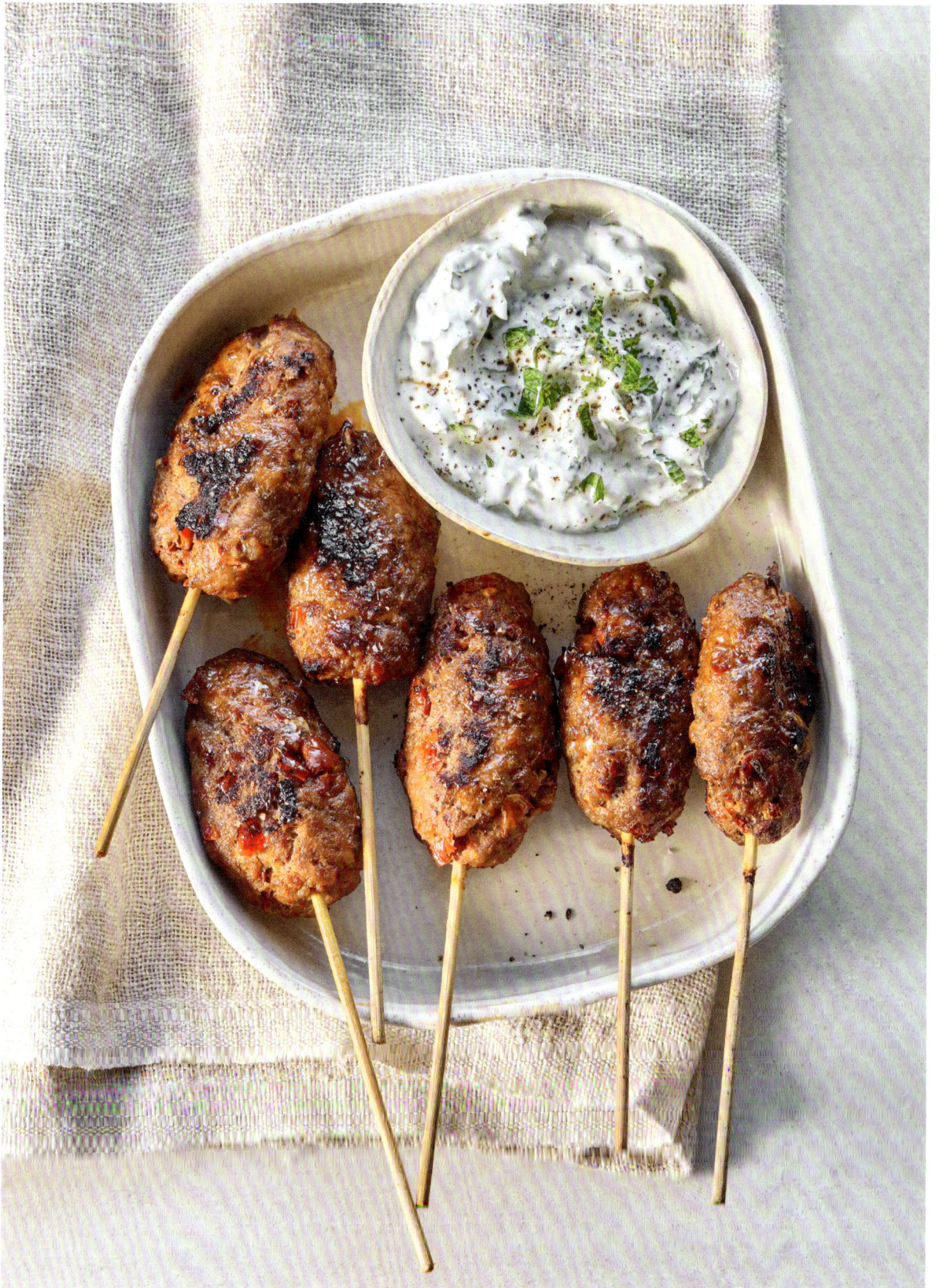

PEANUT-ROASTED CHICKEN IN ROMAINE BOATS

MAKES
4

PREP TIME
25 MINS,
PLUS MARINATING

COOK TIME
20 MINS

30g (1oz) 100 per cent peanut butter

15ml (1 tablespoon) low-salt soy sauce

10g (¼oz) powdered sweetener,
  or honey

10ml (2 teaspoons) sesame oil

1 teaspoon rice vinegar, or apple cider
  vinegar

1 teaspoon garlic purée

1 teaspoon grated fresh root ginger

½ teaspoon chilli flakes

500g (1lb 2oz) boneless, skinless
  chicken breasts, cut into
  bite-sized pieces

sea salt flakes and freshly ground
  black pepper

To serve

12–16 Little Gem lettuce leaves

10g (¼oz) chopped unsalted peanuts

fresh coriander

grated carrot

finely sliced spring onions

MEAT

Prepare for a taste explosion. Marinate the chicken overnight to limit preparation time the following day. This is packed with protein and flavour and is succulent and satisfying. Adjust the seasoning according to your preferences.

1 Whisk together the peanut butter, soy sauce, sweetener or honey, sesame oil, rice vinegar, garlic purée, ginger, chilli flakes, salt and pepper in a mixing bowl. Add the chicken pieces and toss to evenly coat. Leave to marinate for at least 15 minutes.

2 Preheat the oven to 200°C (400°F), Gas Mark 6.

3 Place the marinated chicken pieces on a baking sheet lined with nonstick baking paper, making sure that they are separated and evenly spaced. Roast for 15–20 minutes or until cooked through. Leave to cool slightly.

4 To assemble, divide the chicken among the lettuce leaves. Scatter with chopped peanuts and some coriander, carrot and spring onions, then serve immediately.

PER SERVING	
NET CARBS	6.5G
FIBRE	2.3G
PROTEIN	33G
FAT	9.4G
KCAL	247

RECIPE TIP

You can use another type of lettuce, such as Romaine, if you prefer – just ensure the filling is contained within each leaf so you can hold it. Try wrapping each assembled leaf in some kitchen foil for a lunchbox or picnic.

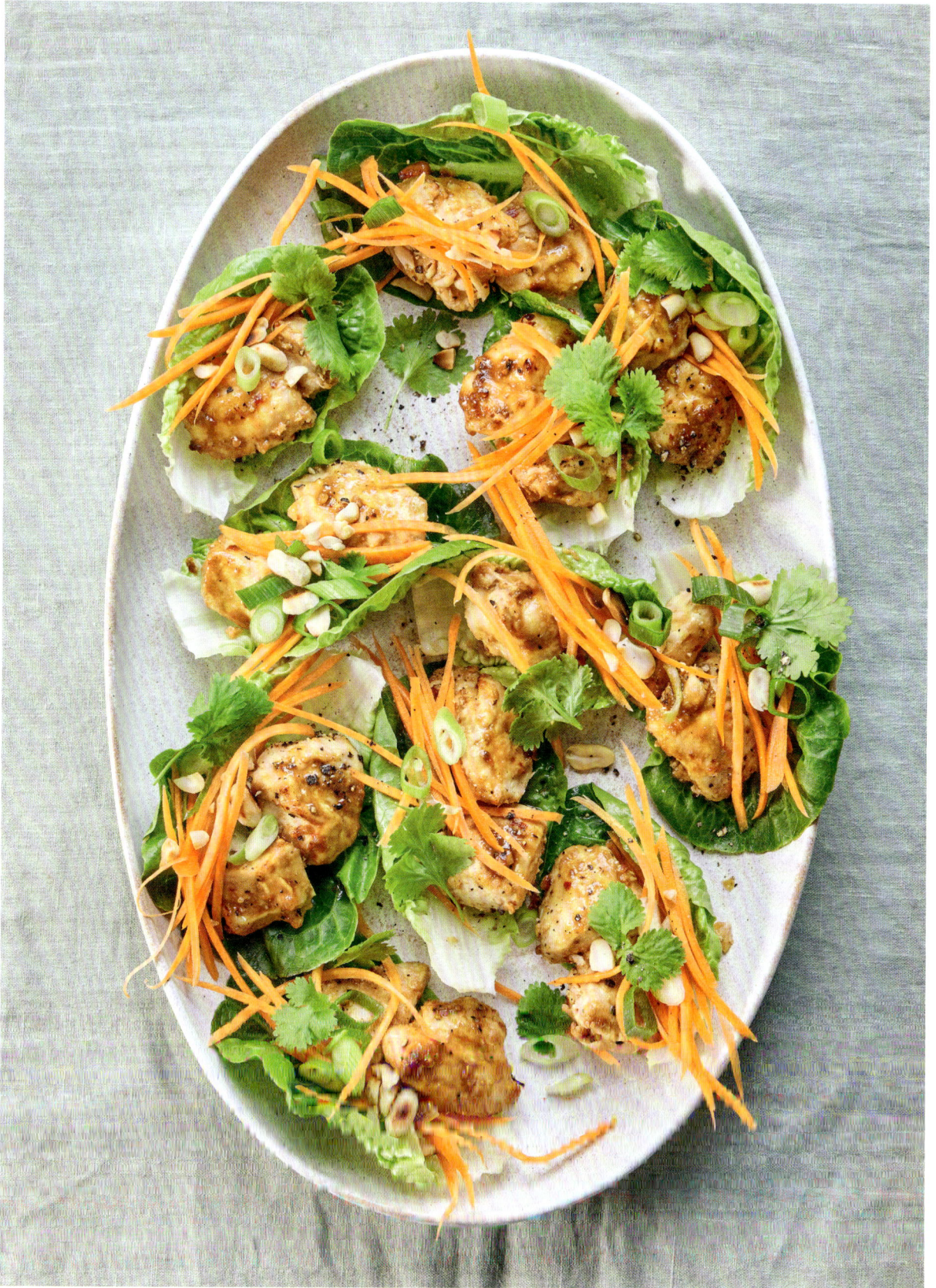

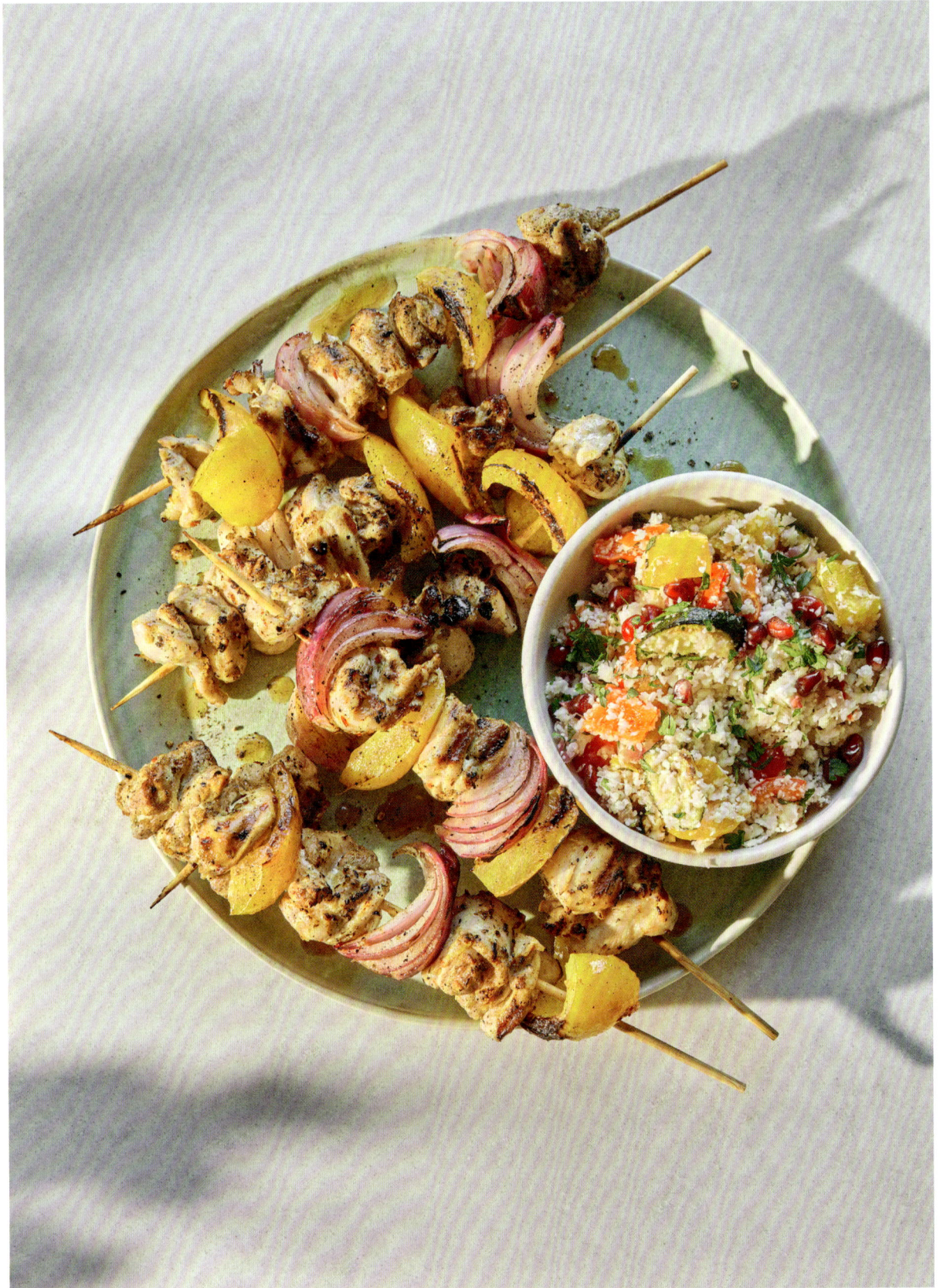

MARINATED CHICKEN KEBABS

2 garlic cloves, very finely chopped or finely grated

finely grated zest and juice of 1 lemon

110ml (8 tablespoons) olive oil

1 teaspoon dried oregano

1 teaspoon chilli flakes

1 red onion, sliced

1 yellow pepper, sliced

500g (1lb 2oz) skinless boneless chicken thighs, cut into large cubes

sea salt flakes and freshly ground black pepper

PER SERVING	
NET CARBS	5.4G
FIBRE	2.5G
PROTEIN	33G
FAT	25G
KCAL	383

I created this recipe during lockdown and developed it in cooking classes I gave over Zoom. My students were from all over the world, so the ingredients had to be simple as people were joining from countries where some items just didn't exist. Often, we'd discuss suitable alternatives that were available for them. I hope that you, too, will be able to improvise and personalize these recipes: sometimes it is difficult to find certain ingredients, or you don't like some of them, but if you are happy to try to find suitable swaps, you will still succeed!

Please allow for the marinating time to let the flavours infuse. If you are fortunate enough to have a barbecue, these kebabs cook beautifully on that.

1 Whisk together the garlic, lemon zest and juice, olive oil, oregano, chilli, salt and pepper in a small bowl. Add the red onion, yellow pepper and chicken and toss to ensure everything is well coated. Cover and refrigerate for a few hours (2–4 hours would be ideal). Remove from the refrigerator and allow to marinate for at least 30 minutes at room temperature before cooking.

2 Meanwhile, place 8–10 wooden skewers into water for at least 20 minutes (no need to follow this step if using metal skewers).

3 Once the chicken has been marinated, alternate threading pieces of chicken, pepper and onion on the skewers, leaving a small space between each piece to allow the heat to move freely and cook everything evenly.

4 Heat a gas grill or griddle to medium-high heat. Grill the chicken for 10–12 minutes, turning occasionally, until thoroughly cooked. If you would prefer to roast, preheat the oven to 180°C (350°F), Gas Mark 4 and place the skewers on a baking sheet. Bake for 20–25 minutes until thoroughly cooked.

RECIPE TIP

I recommend serving these with a side dish of my Cauliflower 'Couscous' with Roasted Vegetables (see page 121).

MEAT

COTTAGE PIE
WITH A SWEDE AND CHEDDAR TOPPING

MEAT

SERVES
6

PREP TIME
20 MINS

COOK TIME
1 HOUR 20 MINS

For the filling

2 tablespoons olive oil

150g (5½oz) onions, finely chopped

150g (5½oz) red pepper, deseeded and chopped

600g (1lb 5oz) minced beef

3 garlic cloves, finely sliced

1½ teaspoons smoked paprika

1 beef stock cube, crumbled

1 teaspoon ground coriander

½ teaspoon ground cumin

2 x 400g (14oz) cans of tomatoes

sea salt flakes and freshly ground black pepper

For the topping

600g (1lb 5oz) swede, peeled and chopped into large chunks

knob of unsalted butter

80g (2¾oz) Cheddar cheese, grated

PER SERVING	
NET CARBS	15G
FIBRE	6.1G
PROTEIN	35G
FAT	21G
KCAL	402

The ultimate comfort food and the perfect centrepiece for any family meal. The grated swede and Cheddar topping is a fantastic alternative to potato and the swede adds taste and texture. Swede is a most underrated vegetable, but it is especially brilliant for those living with diabetes due to its low carb content. It is best served with greens, such as broccoli and kale, to add a boost of fibre.

This dish can be portioned up and frozen, or chilled and enjoyed over a couple of days.

1 Make the filling. Heat the olive oil in a large saucepan over a medium heat. Add the onions and pepper and fry until soft. Once softened, add the beef and stir, breaking it up with a wooden spoon, until browned.

2 Add the garlic and cook for another couple of minutes before adding the smoked paprika, stock cube, coriander and cumin. Stir and cook for 3–4 minutes, but do not let the mixture stick. (If it starts to stick, reduce the heat and mix in 1 tablespoon water.) Add the tomatoes, then fill one of the cans with water and pour that in, too.

3 Bring to the boil for a few minutes, then reduce the heat and simmer uncovered for about 30 minutes until thickened. If it seems too thin, return to a high heat and let it reduce until thick. Season with salt and pepper to taste and spoon into a flameproof baking dish.

4 Preheat the oven to 180°C (350°F), Gas Mark 4.

5 Meanwhile, prepare the topping. Cook the swede in a pan of boiling salted water for 10 minutes until tender, then drain and set aside. When the swede is cool enough to handle, coarsely grate it using a box grater; then toss in the butter and Cheddar and season. Stir until the butter is melted and everything is combined.

6 Carefully spoon the swede mixture over the beef and place in the oven for 25 minutes.

7 Preheat the grill. Place the pie under the hot grill for a final 5 minutes until the topping turns golden brown and the filling is piping hot. Allow to cool for a few minutes before serving.

EGG-FRIED CAULIFLOWER 'RICE'

SERVES
4

PREP TIME
15 MINS

COOK TIME
15 MINS

400g (14oz) cauliflower florets, tough central stalk removed

2 teaspoons coconut oil

1 red onion, finely chopped

2 garlic cloves, finely chopped

½ small green chilli, deseeded and finely chopped

1 green pepper, finely chopped

500g (1lb 2oz) skinless boneless chicken thighs, chopped

1 teaspoon garam masala

2 teaspoons ground cumin

1 teaspoon ground coriander

1 vegetable stock cube, or a generous pinch of sea salt flakes

2 tablespoons water

1 large egg

2 handfuls of spinach

handful of chopped fresh coriander, plus more to serve

sea salt flakes and freshly ground black pepper

To serve (optional)

lime wedges

low-salt soy sauce

If you live with diabetes and are anything like me, your blood sugars will resent every grain of rice consumed, making meal times very challenging. However, this dish is a joy to eat and will not leave you feeling unwell. It has everything you want from egg-fried rice, but without the rice! Instead, cauliflower is used as an alternative; please do not roll your eyes, just try it! Cauliflower 'rice' complements the dish, giving you the texture of regular rice and absorbing flavours in much the same way.

1 Place the chopped cauliflower in a blender and pulse-blend to a rice-like consistency.

2 Melt the coconut oil in a large saucepan over a medium heat, add the onion, garlic, chilli and green pepper and fry until soft and golden.

3 Add the chicken and fry it off for a couple of minutes before adding the spices, stock cube and a pinch of cracked black pepper. Cook for a few minutes.

4 Add the cauliflower and measured water and cook for a further 5 minutes, stirring occasionally. Add the egg and spinach and stir constantly for 1 minute. Add the chopped coriander.

5 Serve immediately, with a lime wedge and a splash of soy sauce, if you like.

MEAT

PER SERVING	
NET CARBS	12G
FIBRE	4.1G
PROTEIN	17G
FAT	16G
KCAL	356

RECIPE TIP

If you would like to make this a vegetarian dish, leave out the chicken and replace it with a plant-based alternative such as tofu or Quorn. You might also like to try king prawns or a firm white fish fillet such as cod, which both work beautifully well.

PROTEIN PIZZA

SERVES

3 / MAKES 6 LARGE SLICES

PREP TIME

10 MINS

COOK TIME

20 MINS, OR 40 MINUTES IF
MAKING THE TOMATO SAUCE

*For the sauce (optional, makes
enough for 2 Protein pizzas)*

400g (14oz) can of tomatoes

1 teaspoon dried parsley

1 teaspoon dried oregano

1 teaspoon dried thyme

1 teaspoon paprika

sea salt flakes and freshly ground
    black pepper (optional)

For the base

280g (10oz) skinless boneless chicken
    thighs, chopped

90g (3¼oz) grated mozzarella

45g (1½oz) ground almonds, or ground
    flaxseed / linseed

1 teaspoon mixed herbs (optional)

*For the toppings (these are some
favourite combinations, but use
whatever you prefer)*

goat's cheese, red onion and spinach

artichokes, yellow pepper and red
    onion

ham, pineapple and black olives

mushrooms, red pepper and
    roasted garlic

FOR 2 SLICES (NO TOPPINGS)	
NET CARBS	8.8G
FIBRE	4.2G
PROTEIN	36G
FAT	25G
KCAL	409

Believe it or not, this pizza base is made from chicken! It is so tasty, holds together beautifully and is always a crowd-pleaser: a great dish for sharing with friends or family with a side salad. You could serve it for a Friday night fakeaway, perhaps with Smoky Sweet Potato Fries on the side (see page 124).

1   For the sauce, tip the tomatoes into a saucepan over high heat. Bring to a bubble, then reduce the heat to a simmer. Add a pinch of salt and all the herbs and spices and simmer until the sauce has thickened. Set aside to cool.

2   Preheat the oven to 180°C (350°F), Gas Mark 4.

3   Place the chicken in a food processor and pulse-blend until a sticky mince. This might take a couple of minutes. Add the mozzarella, ground almonds, mixed herbs, if using, and season. Pulse until combined.

4   Grab a silicone baking sheet or a sheet of nonstick baking paper. Press the chicken mixture into a large rectangular or circular pizza base shape, either with your hands (wear disposable gloves if you like), or roll it out between 2 sheets of baking parchment. The thinner you can make this, the better, but do ensure there are no holes. Place the pizza base on the baking sheet or sheet of nonstick baking paper.

5   Pop the pizza base in the oven and bake for 10 minutes until firm and cooked. Remove from the oven, spread with the tomato sauce, if using, and add your chosen toppings.

6   Reduce the oven temperature to 170°C (340°F), Gas Mark 3½ and bake for a further 8–10 minutes until the toppings are cooked (you might need to adjust this time depending on your toppings).

7   Remove from the oven and serve straightaway. Or allow to fully cool, cover and chill to enjoy cold. Eat within 24 hours.

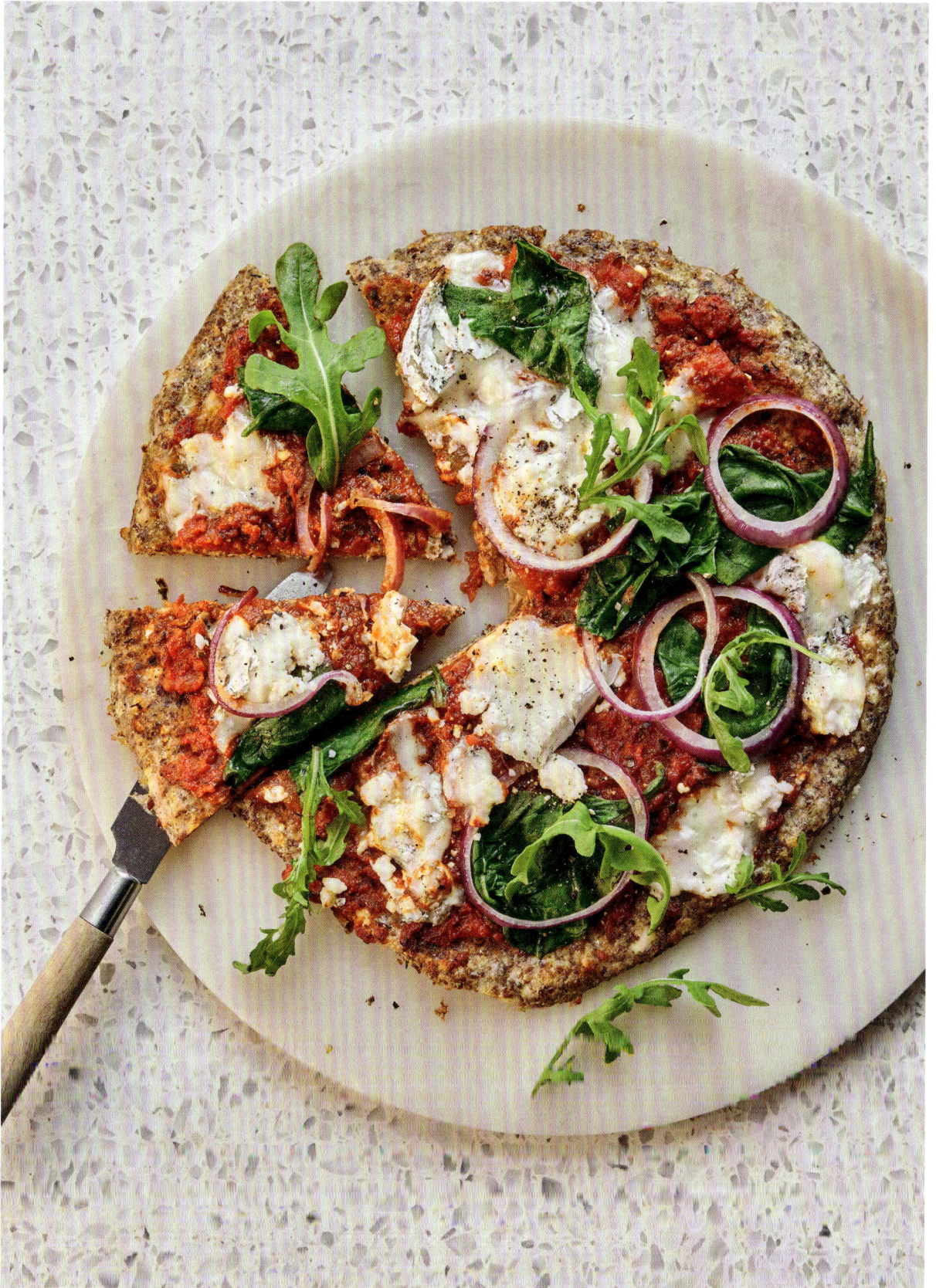

SPICY BANG BANG CHICKEN SALAD

SERVES
2

PREP TIME
10 MINS

COOK TIME
10 MINS

200g (7oz) crunchy salad bag mix

60g (2¼oz) cherry tomatoes, halved

50g (1¾oz) cucumber, finely sliced

50g (1¾oz) purple cabbage, thinly sliced

1 carrot, grated

40g (1½oz) toasted cashew nuts

1 teaspoon olive oil

350g (12oz) boneless, skinless,chicken breast, chopped

1 teaspoon chilli powder

1 teaspoon smoked paprika

1 teaspoon ground cumin

1 teaspoon mustard seeds

1 teaspoon garlic purée

1 teaspoon nigella seeds

2 tablespoons water

sea salt and cracked black pepper

For the dressing

40g (1½oz) yogurt

2 tablespoon sriracha

1 teaspoon lime juice

This is a taste sensation and the perfect dish for using up leftover roast chicken. When chicken is seasoned perfectly, there really is nothing better! Cook the chicken in the spices and place in an airtight container for lunch the next day.

1 Place the leaves in a large bowl with the tomatoes, cucumber, purple cabbage and carrot.

2 Place a nonstick frying pan over a medium heat and add the cashew nuts. After 1 minute, shake the pan to ensure the nuts are toasted evenly. After another couple of minutes you will be able to smell the toasted aroma. Remove from the heat and set aside in a bowl.

3 Return the pan to the heat, add the olive oil and fry the chicken for 2 minutes. Add the chilli, paprika, cumin and mustard seeds and continue to fry for a further 2–3 minutes. As the chicken turns golden brown, add the garlic purée and nigella seeds and cook for a further minute. Add the measured water to deglaze the pan, stir the chicken and cook for a further 2 minutes. Once the chicken is fully cooked, season with salt and pepper and transfer to a bowl.

4 In a separate small bowl, stir together the yogurt, sriracha and lime juice.

5 Add the warm chicken and toasted nuts to the salad bowl and cover with the spicy dressing. Toss together thoroughly and divide evenly between 2 serving bowls.

PER SERVING	
NET CARBS	21G
FIBRE	7.5G
PROTEIN	54G
FAT	20G
KCAL	495

RECIPE TIP As with any salads, if there are ingredients you don't like, then simply leave them out or substitute them for another low-starch vegetable (see the list on page 78).

MEAT

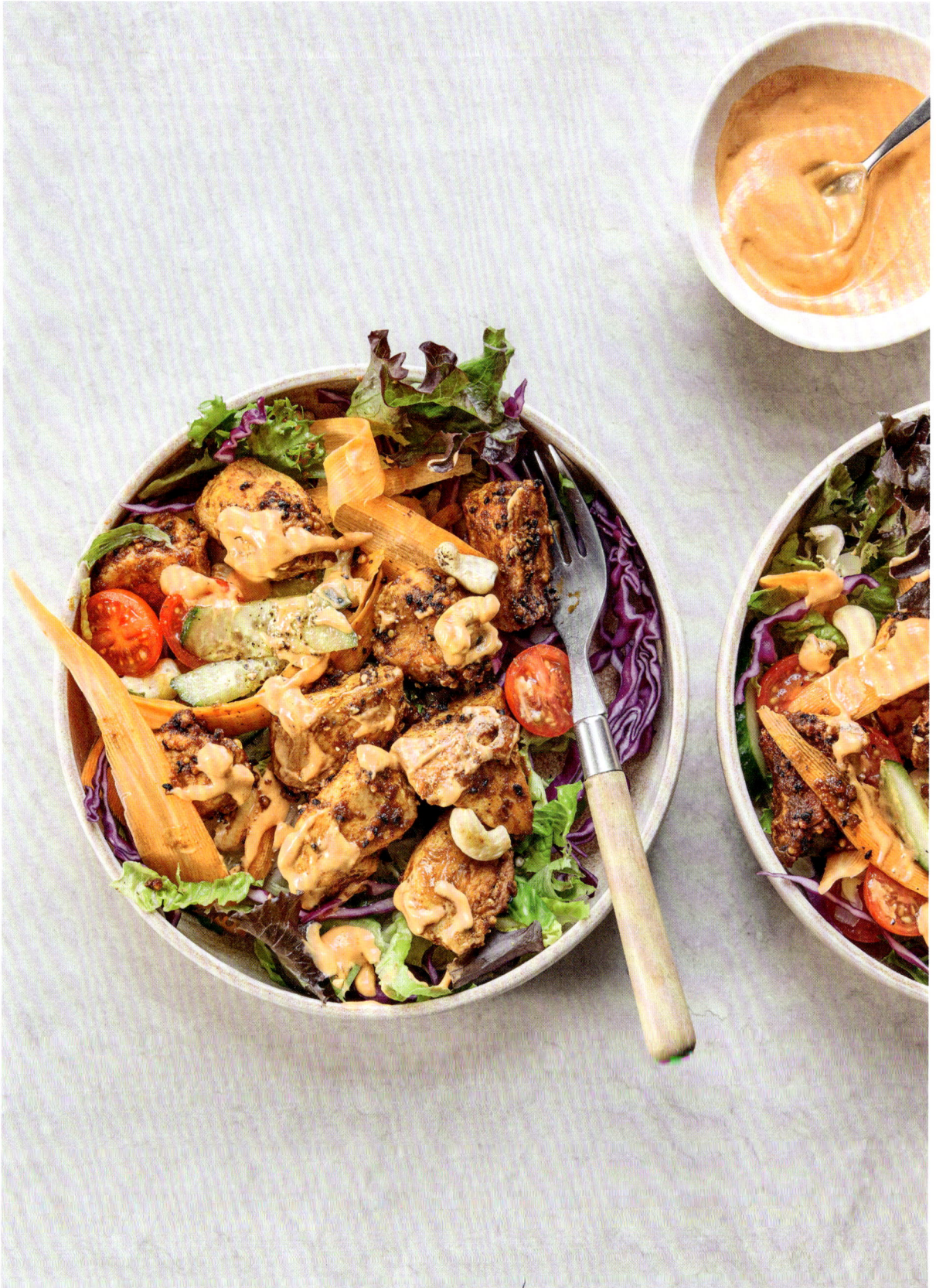

Step-by-step roast dinner

Sundays back home in Wales – as for so many UK families – always included a roast, a walk and the dreaded homework!

The preparations for our roast dinners started before I had even got out of bed. I could hear the clanging of pans, the tap filling them with water, potatoes and apples being peeled and chopped for roasting and for crumble. My dad was in charge of the meat. My brother and I would set the table, fill the water glasses and, once everything was made, we would all sit down together. We would talk about the week gone by and make plans for the week ahead. Pudding was often plum crumble, which we loved as it meant we could count their stones. 'Tinker, tailor, soldier, sailor...' went the old rhyme.

This was before smart phones became a permanent feature. Nowadays, many such conversations around the table have been lost. We have all seen how addictive phones can be. We have all watched people in restaurants not engaging with each other over a meal, but rather engaging with someone else somewhere else, through a screen. Whether it be work or friends or family, we are contactable at any time. This goes for how we are able to get hold of food, too: if we live in a town or city, we can have fast food at our door within minutes at the press of a button.

We are communicating less and we are less aware of what we are eating. Because of multiple screens on the go all the time, excessive calories can be consumed without even thinking about it. So pause, take a breath, put the screen down and engage with those around you at mealtimes.

A weekly roast dinner is an opportunity to take some time away from your busy life. To prepare your meat. To decide how you will serve your vegetables. Perhaps you'll roast some and blanch, boil or steam others. To make a dessert. To set lots of timers, so everything happens at the right time.

Once everything is cooked, you can sit down, plate up and enjoy the food you've made, because it has taken you time and effort and because you deserve it. Granted, the washing-up is not such fun, but it is just some further quiet time away from the busy-ness of life... and more time away from the phone, or mindlessly snacking on the leftovers. After that, try to follow the tradition of going for a Sunday walk, if you can. If you live with diabetes, walking between meals, or a walk after a meal, not only aids digestion but also helps with insulin sensitivity.

And don't worry: once you have conquered your first roast dinner, you will be able to make the next seamlessly. Don't forget that any leftovers, such as meat or vegetables, can go into a curry, a frittata or a quick omelette.

How to keep calories low

Use an olive oil spray for meat and vegetables.

Consider steaming, boiling or blanching vegetables.

Opt for low-starch vegetables to keep both calories and carbs lower (see page 78 for a list).

Remember that lean meats such as chicken or turkey contain less saturated fat than beef or lamb.

Be adventurous with cooking processes and add seasonings such as herbs and spices for added flavour (see page 23 for tips).

Making your own accompaniments – such as Yorkshire puddings (see page 168) and stuffing – will reduce the fat and salt content.

Have a fruit-based dessert with a simple crumble topping (see page 201) and opt for a small portion of Greek yogurt flavoured with sugar-free vanilla extract, rather than cream or custard.

ROAST CHICKEN
WITH LEMON, RED ONION AND LEEK

SERVES
3

PREP TIME
10 MINS

COOK TIME
60 MINS

2 tablespoons olive oil

200g (7oz) red onion, sliced into
  6 wedges through the root

200g (7oz) leeks, sliced

1 lemon, sliced

540g (1lb 4oz) bone-in chicken thighs
  or drumsticks

1 teaspoon dried parsley

1 teaspoon dried rosemary

sea salt flakes and cracked black
  pepper

PER SERVING	
NET CARBS	6.6G
FIBRE	2.7G
PROTEIN	35G
FAT	23G
KCAL	376

A dish that combines a lot of delicious flavours. You can use any cuts of chicken, but a combination of thighs and drumsticks are not only more flavourful than breast, but are inexpensive and work incredibly well when feeding a few people. This is a versatile and easy to prepare dish. Chicken is a lean source of protein and is low in saturated fat, which makes it great for weight management, while also providing a nourishing and filling meal.

1 Preheat the oven to 190°C (375°F), Gas Mark 5.

2 Put the olive oil in a baking dish. Add the onion, leeks and lemon, arranging them evenly. Place the chicken on top and rub with the olive oil in the dish. Season with the dried parsley, rosemary, salt and pepper.

3 Roast for 25 minutes, then give the dish a shake to make sure the chicken and vegetables are evenly cooked, basting the chicken in any juices at the same time.

4 Once the chicken has been roasting for 50 minutes in total, increase the oven temperature to 200°C (400°F), Gas Mark 6 and roast for a further 10 minutes to crisp up the skin.

5 Remove from the oven and ensure the chicken is cooked through. You can either do this with a meat thermometer (it should read 74°C / 165°F), or pierce the thickest part of the chicken with a knife to check the juices run clear. If it's not quite ready, cook for 5 minutes longer, then check again.

6 Serve immediately with any other accompaniments, or place in a warming oven until everything is ready.

RECIPE TIP
Pour the chicken juices into a gravy boat, add 1 tablespoon organic low-salt gravy granules and top with some boiling water. Stir together to combine and serve the gravy with the chicken.

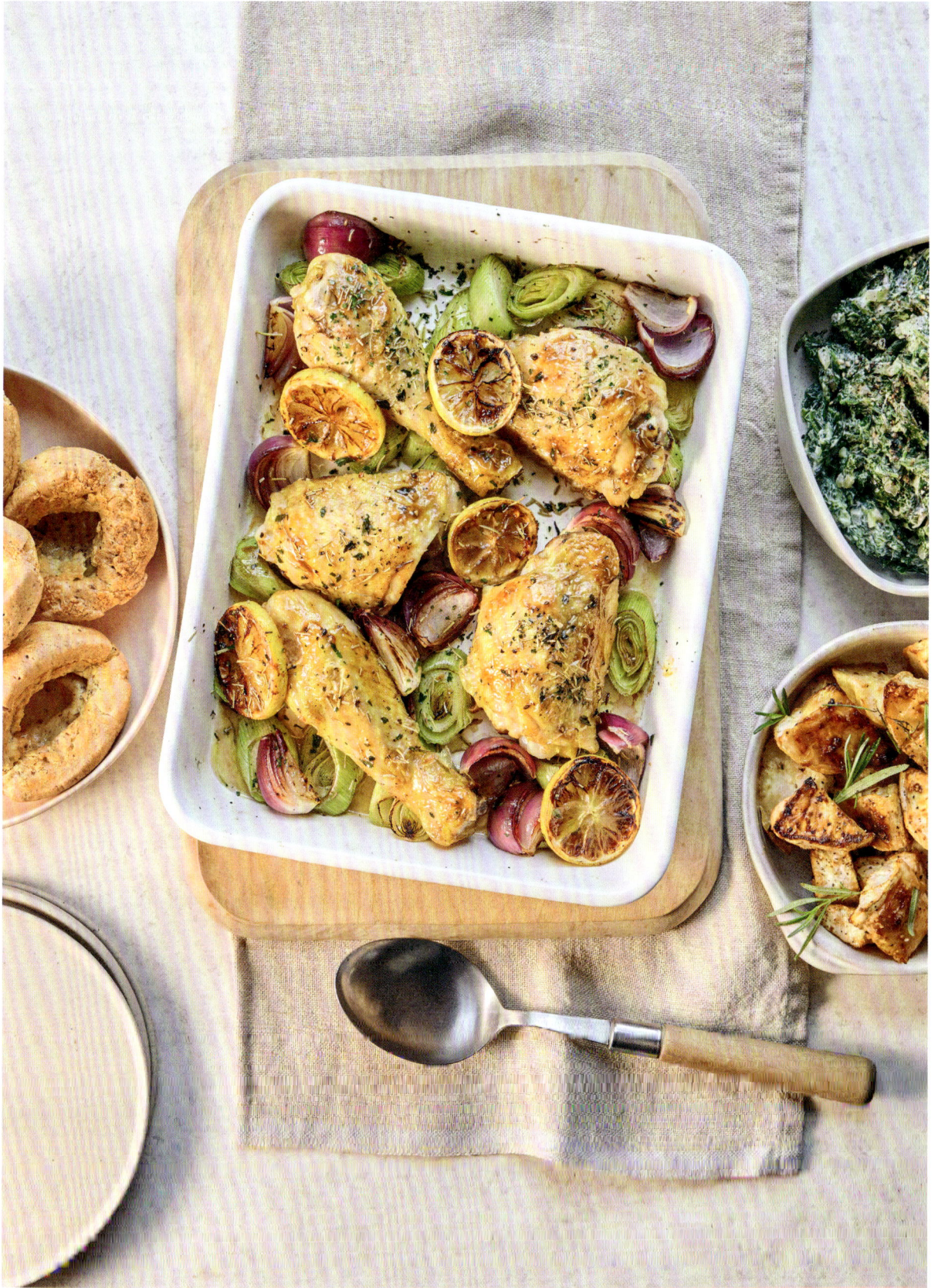

LOWER-CARB YORKSHIRE PUDDINGS

SERVES
6–8

PREP TIME
5 MINS

COOK TIME
20–25 MINS

goose fat, or beef dripping (or see recipe introduction)

2 large eggs

55ml (2fl oz) milk (full-fat milk, semi-skimmed milk or almond milk)

55ml (2fl oz) double cream

35g (1¼oz) arrowroot (see below)

15g (½oz) ground flaxseeds / linseeds or ground almonds

PER SERVING	
NET CARBS	5.5G
FIBRE	0.8G
PROTEIN	3.3G
FAT	12G
KCAL	149

It is hard to believe that, by just changing a few ingredients, Yorkshire puddings can be a healthier choice – this recipe creates the same taste and texture as the traditional carb-filled variety. Goose fat is stocked in supermarkets all year round and you'll need that, or beef dripping, to make these well, as it has such a high smoking point. Please be aware that, if you choose to use light olive oil instead, it has a lower smoking point so it could burn. These sit perfectly alongside a Sunday roast, or the batter can be used to pour over a batch of sausages to create a delightful toad-in-the-hole.

1 Preheat the oven to 200°C (400°F), Gas Mark 6.

2 Grab a solid cupcake or muffin mould and place ½ teaspoon of fat into each hollow. Place into the hottest part of the oven for 5–10 minutes to heat up.

3 Meanwhile, make the batter. Put the eggs, milk and cream in a bowl and whisk together. Add the arrowroot and flaxseed and whisk.

4 Being very careful when moving the extremely hot fat out of the oven, pour about a 2.5cm (1 inch) depth of batter into each mould (you need each to be about half full). Carefully place in the hottest part of the oven and cook for 15 minutes. Keep checking every 5 or so minutes until they have risen and are golden brown. Depending on your oven, your puddings might require an extra 5 minutes. Do not open the oven, or they will go flat.

5 Remove once they are risen and a golden brown colour. Serve immediately.

RECIPE TIP

In this recipe the arrowroot is an essential ingredient, so don't be tempted to leave it out or substitute it. I buy inexpensive arrowroot powder from the baking aisle of big supermarkets, where it's generally found next to baking powder and in a similar pot. You can buy it online or in most health food shops, too.

ROASTED CELERIAC AND ROSEMARY ROASTIES

SERVES

2

PREP TIME
10 MINS

COOK TIME
40 MINS

2 tablespoons light olive oil

700g (1lb 9oz) celeriac, peeled

1 teaspoon sea salt flakes

4 teaspoons rosemary leaves

2 teaspoons garlic purée

PER SERVING	
NET CARBS	9.3G
FIBRE	13G
PROTEIN	4.7G
FAT	14G
KCAL	210

If you miss roast potatoes, these roasties with rosemary and garlic will fill that gap. Celeriac is a root vegetable with a mild flavour and is a perfect potato substitute. It is similar to parsnip in texture and taste, but smells like celery! It is great roasted, steamed, in soups, as fries or mashed. You can enjoy it roasted alongside other vegetables and partner it with a succulent steak or a Sunday roast.

1 Preheat the oven to 180°C (350°F), Gas Mark 4. Drizzle the olive oil into a deep baking dish to cover the bottom and place in the oven to heat for 10 minutes.

2 Cut the celeriac into roast potato-sized chunks. The thickness is up to you, but don't make them too big, or they will take too long to cook.

3 Carefully remove the baking dish from the oven and add the celeriac, turning the chunks over to coat in the oil. Add the sea salt flakes, then bake for 20 minutes.

4 After 20 minutes, remove the dish from the oven, turn the chunks over to ensure they cook evenly. Add the rosemary, stir in the garlic purée and bake for a further 20 minutes until the roasties are tender and the rosemary fragrant. Remove from the oven and serve immediately.

CREAMED SPINACH

SERVES
4

PREP TIME
5 MINS

COOK TIME
10 MINS

500g (1lb 2oz) frozen chopped spinach

20g (¾oz) unsalted butter

1 onion, finely chopped

100g (3½oz) cream cheese

about 20ml (4 teaspoons) milk
(any milk is fine here)

ground nutmeg, to taste

sea salt flakes

PER SERVING	
NET CARBS	4.5G
FIBRE	4.6G
PROTEIN	6G
FAT	13G
KCAL	171

A perfect accompaniment to a roast dinner that's quick and easy to make. Frozen spinach is fantastic value in the supermarket, so do get some if you have space in your freezer. Cream cheese adds a tasty richness to this leafy green veg..

1 Defrost the spinach (it is best defrosted in the refrigerator overnight). Transfer to a sieve and press firmly to squeeze out any excess moisture.

2 Melt the butter in a large saucepan and cook the onion for a few minutes over a high heat until soft and translucent. Reduce the heat and stir in the cream cheese. Add the drained spinach and combine all the ingredients together.

3 Add a little milk to achieve your preferred consistency. Season with a little sea salt and nutmeg, to taste. Transfer to a serving dish and take to the table.

RECIPE TIP

You can make this up to 24 hours in advance: just cover and refrigerate. When ready to serve, return it to a pan and reheat over a medium heat until piping hot. Add a splash of milk to loosen, if needed.

CAULIFLOWER MASH

SERVES

3

PREP TIME

5 MINS

COOK TIME

20 MINS

1 large cauliflower

1 tablespoon unsalted butter

2 tablespoons soured cream

sea salt flakes and freshly ground
   black pepper

PER SERVING	
NET CARBS	12.2G
FIBRE	4.8G
PROTEIN	7.2G
FAT	7.6G
KCAL	142

When food makes you feel good, you want to keep eating it! This recipe will prove to you that cauliflower mash is a worthy alternative topping for a pie and it works with stews, sausages or a roast dinner. It is low in calories and incredibly low in carbs, but it remains comforting, nourishing and filling. Try serving potato mash alongside cauliflower mash: you may be surprised to see which one is the most popular. Making the swap might feel like an impossible hurdle, but give it a go. You won't be disappointed.

1 Remove any leaves from your cauliflower (save them for a stock or soup). Break it into florets and chop up the stalk. Pop the florets and stalk in a deep saucepan over a high heat, just cover with water, then cover with a lid. Bring to the boil, then reduce the heat to a simmer and cook for 15 minutes, or until tender and easy to mash.

2 Drain well and place into a mixing bowl or the bowl of a blender. Add the butter, soured cream, pepper and a pinch of sea salt. Either use a potato masher or purée in a blender until smooth and creamy.

VARIATIONS

Cheesy mash
Place the mash in a small ovenproof bowl, top with 50g (1¾oz) grated Parmesan cheese, then pop under a preheated grill for 10 minutes until bubbling and golden.

Topping for a pie
Try cooked cauliflower mashed with another low-starch vegetable such as cooked broccoli, or finely shred some cabbage and add it to the cauliflower 2 minutes before the end of the cooking time. Add a pinch of sea salt, 1 tablespoon double cream and 1 tablespoon unsalted butter, then top with 2 tablespoons ground almonds and 1 tablespoon chopped chives and you'll have a delicious topping for a stew or pie mix (this would work brilliantly for a fish pie or cottage pie, see pages 144 and 158).

CHICKPEA FLATBREADS

MAKES
4 PITTA BREAD-SIZED
FLATBREADS

2 teaspoons baking powder

1 tablespoon apple cider vinegar

90g (3¼oz) Greek yogurt

1 teaspoon olive oil, plus more to cook

90g (3¼oz) chickpea flour, plus more
   to dust

1 teaspoon xanthan gum, ideally, or
   ground flaxseed / linseed, milled
   chia seed, or arrowroot

sea salt flakes

PER FLATBREAD	
NET CARBS	13G
FIBRE	2.9G
PROTEIN	6.5G
FAT	6.7G
KCAL	146

RECIPE TIP

These can be made in advance
and frozen. To cook frozen
Chickpea flatbreads, completely
defrost them, then place in a hot
frying pan over a medium heat
and carefully reheat both sides to
piping hot before serving.

PREP TIME
10 MINS

COOK TIME
6–8 MINS, WITH 2 FRYING PANS,
12–16 MINUTES WITH 1 FRYING
PAN

These are quick to make, but they contain fewer than half the calories
and carbs of a wheat-based flatbread. They are fantastic with curries,
soups and stews; great for dipping and dunking! Chickpea flour,
also known as gram flour, has become mainstream over the last few
years and can be picked up in any big supermarket or health food
shop alongside other flours. It is rich in protein and dietary fibre and
absolutely perfect to serve with Roasted Paneer and Tomato Curry
with Cauliflower 'Rice', Chickpea Dal, or Marinated Chicken Kebabs
(see pages 126, 129 and 157).

1 Spoon the baking powder and apple cider vinegar into a mixing bowl
   and allow it to fizz. Once it stops fizzing, whisk in the Greek yogurt and
   olive oil.

2 Fold in the chickpea flour, xanthan gum and a pinch of salt and mix
   with a spatula until you have a thick dough.

3 Break into 4 balls of about 50g (1¾oz) each and mould each into an
   oval shape. Roll out between 2 lightly floured pieces of nonstick baking
   paper to about 5mm (¼ inch) thick.

4 Place a frying pan – or use 2, to cook these more quickly – over a
   medium heat and spray sparingly with olive oil. Transfer a flatbread to
   a pan and cook for 3–4 minutes, then flip and cook on the other side for
   3–4 minutes.

5 Once cooked, remove from the frying pan and wrap in a tea towel to
   keep warm and flexible while you quickly cook the other flatbreads
   and serve as soon as possible. Or you can leave them to thoroughly
   cool, then store in an airtight container at room temperature for up to
   3 days.

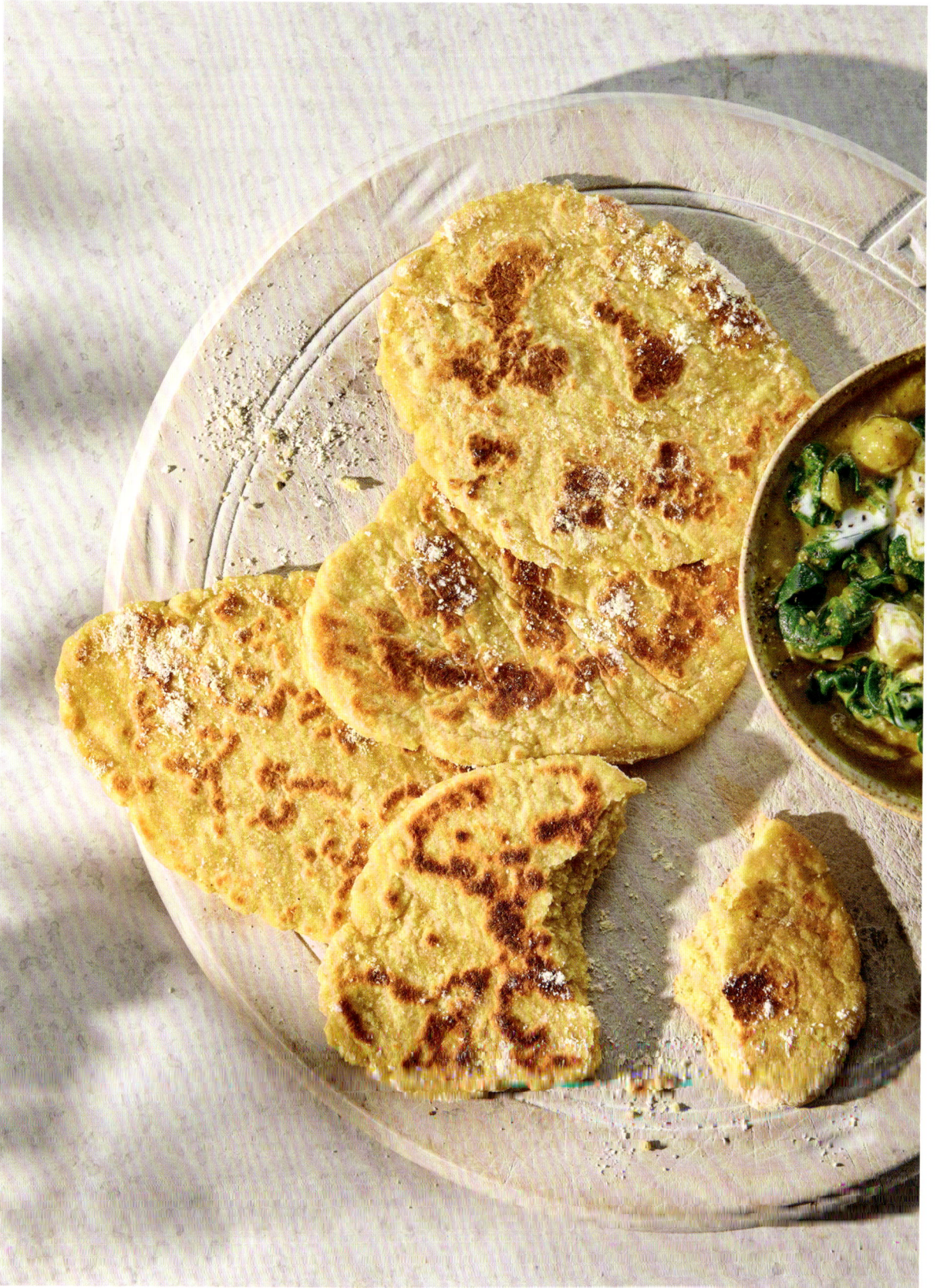

FIVE-INGREDIENT FIBRE BREAD

MAKES
1 LOAF / 18 SLICES

PREP TIME
10 MINS

COOK TIME
25 MINS

2 tablespoons olive oil, plus more for the tin

300g (10½oz) ground brown flaxseeds / linseeds (or see below)

2 teaspoons baking powder

5 large eggs

4 tablespoons water

sea salt (optional)

PER SLICE	
NET CARBS	<1G
FIBRE	4.7G
PROTEIN	4G
FAT	10G
KCAL	118

RECIPE TIP

If you want to save money and you have a high-powered blender, or a blender with a nut milling function, or even a coffee grinder, you can consider bulk-buying flaxseed / linseed in 1kg (2lb 4oz) bags. Blend it to a coarse flour, then store in an airtight jar and use whenever required; it will keep for up to 4 months.

You can also buy ready-milled flaxseed / linseed, though it is more expensive than buying the whole seed variety and grinding it yourself.

A simple brown bread, full of fibre and protein, low in carbs and with only 118 kcal in a slice: perfect for open sandwiches. Commercially produced shop-bought bread can contain up to 20 ingredients, is ultra-processed and has a high salt content. For many people living with diabetes, eating processed bread is a major problem, because a single slice contains a high amount of carbs, even before you add any fillings or toppings. If you can find the time to make your own bread, you will reap the health benefits. The great thing about this bread is that you can bake it, slice it and freeze it. This way, you will have it in the freezer ready to pop slices straight in the toaster. Serve with a small amount of unsalted butter and homemade jam (see page 184). You will need a 450g (1lb) loaf tin. A silicone tin works well, but a traditional metal tin gives a better crust.

1 Preheat the oven to 180°C (350°F), Gas Mark 4. Oil a 450g (1lb) loaf tin and line it with nonstick baking paper.

2 Place the flaxseeds and baking powder in a deep mixing bowl and combine them. Make a well in the middle of the mixture.

3 In a separate bowl, beat together the eggs, oil and measured water until well-combined and smooth. Add a pinch of salt, if you want.

4 Pour the egg mix into the well and, using a wooden spoon, combine the wet and dry ingredients to form a thick batter. Spoon it into the prepared loaf tin and bake in the middle of the oven for 25 minutes until the bread has risen and formed a solid crust. (If you don't have a fan-assisted oven, this may take a little longer.)

5 Carefully remove the bread and allow to cool on a wire rack. (If you find the bread is stuck to the inside of the tin, it sometimes helps to wait for it to fully cool before removing.)

6 Allow the bread to cool completely before storing in an airtight container. It will keep at room temperature for up to 4 days and in the refrigerator for up to 8 days, or slice and freeze for up to 3 months.

WAYS TO ENJOY FIVF-INGREDIENT FIBRE BREAD

An open sandwich makes a great light lunch, toasted or not. Here are some of my favourite open sandwiches:

TUNA WITH SPRING ONION, WHOLEGRAIN MUSTARD, GREEK YOGURT AND BLACK PEPPER

Take a 145g/5¼oz can of tuna in water or brine and add the drained fish to a bowl with 2 tablespoons low-fat Greek yogurt, 1 finely sliced spring onion, a squeeze of lemon juice, 1 teaspoon wholegrain mustard and a twist of black pepper. Mix together and serve on a slice of bread.

AVOCADO AND 'JAMMY' EGG WITH SEA SALT FLAKES

Peel, pit and finely slice ½ avocado. Lay it on a slice of toasted bread. Cut a Perfect soft-boiled 'jammy' egg (see page 96) in half and place on the avocado. Sprinkle with sea salt flakes and serve.

MIXED ROASTED VEGETABLES WITH CRUMBLED FETA CHEESE

Cut a selection of low-starch vegetables (such as cauliflower, Brussels sprouts, peppers, mushrooms, tomatoes, courgettes, aubergines or red onion, see page 78 for a list) into bite-sized chunks. Place in an ovenproof dish, spray with olive oil, season with a generous amount of salt and black pepper and toss together so the vegetables are evenly covered. Roast in an oven preheated to 180°C (350°F), Gas Mark 4 until fragrant, soft and caramelized at the edges. Allow to cool, then place in an airtight container in the refrigerator for up to 5 days. You can reheat to piping hot if desired. Serve on a slice of toasted bread, using 150g (5½oz) roasted veg and 25g (1oz) crumbled feta cheese.

PEANUT BUTTER WITH RASPBERRIES

Here's a sweet twist on an open sandwich. Peanut butter is very moreish, so try to eat it only occasionally. Spread 1 teaspoon 100 per cent peanut butter on a slice of toasted bread, mash some raspberries on top and add a tiny sprinkle of sea salt flakes. Yum.

BAKES

MACKEREL WITH SHREDDED CABBAGE, CARROT AND SPRING ONION

Canned mackerel is fantastic for this as it is quick, cheaper than fresh fish and readily available. I like to use a 125g (4½oz) can of mackerel in olive oil. Drain, then add it to a bowl with some black pepper and ½ teaspoon wholegrain mustard and mix. Coarsely grate 1 small carrot and add to the mackerel with 40g (1½oz) shredded cabbage, 1 sliced spring onion and 2 teaspoons mayonnaise. Stir, then spread on a slice of toasted bread. Fish is an excellent source of protein and beautifully complements the crunchy slaw.

FIG AND GREEK YOGURT

Spread Greek yogurt on a slice of toasted bread and top with slices of fresh fig. A sprinkle of hemp seeds or toasted pumpkin and sunflower seeds on top would make a lovely addition. If you want to add honey, then please do so – just be mindful of how much you use, as it will affect the carb count and your 'drizzle' of honey will, of course, be different from mine! There are sugar-free syrups on the market, which might work better with your blood sugars, but they are always heavily processed, so take a look at the ingredients before using.

TOAST AND JAM

Toast a slice of bread, spread with a thin layer of butter and top with a layer of my Low-Sugar Blackberry Jam (see page 184).

Eating this takes me straight back to afternoons at home after school, sitting at home watching children's TV with my brother while eating toast and jam. In the background would be a muted clatter from the kitchen where mum was preparing dinner. The food we eat can evoke sentimental memories, especially those from childhood, and still being able to recreate a healthier jam on toast reminiscent of a childhood tea is brilliant: there really is little better.

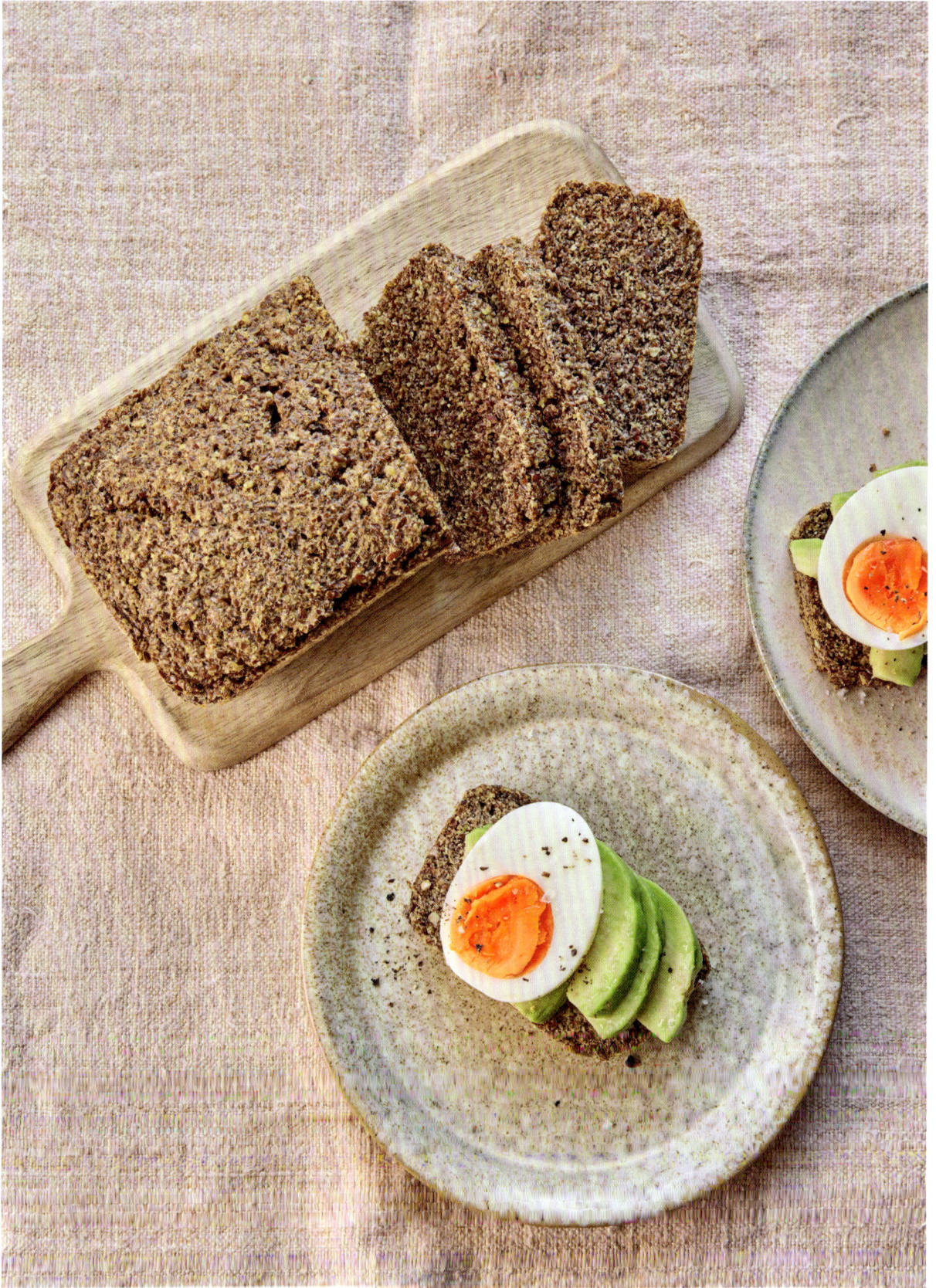

MULTISEED CRACKERS

MAKES
30

PREP TIME
10 MINS

COOK TIME
35–45 MINS

210g (7½oz) mixed seeds

100g (3½oz) milled seeds

7g (¼oz) psyllium husk

1 teaspoon sea salt flakes

1 teaspoon ground cumin

½ teaspoon cumin seeds

1 teaspoon dried thyme

200ml (7fl oz) water

2 tablespoons olive oil

1 tablespoon apple cider vinegar

PER CRACKER	
NET CARBS	1.2G
FIBRE	0.8G
PROTEIN	2.3G
FAT	5.7G
KCAL	66

These are a perfect crunchy, healthy snack as an alternative to highly processed crackers. Try them with some crudités and my Roasted Beetroot Hummus (see pages 66 and 71), or as croutons scattered over a salad or soup, or just on their own. Be mindful of portion control, as they are incredibly moreish. (You can make them, portion them up with 3 per portion and freeze if necessary, to avoid temptation.)

1   Preheat the oven to 170°C (340°F), Gas Mark 3½.

2   Combine all the dry ingredients in a bowl and mix. Separately combine the wet ingredients in a jug.

3   Pour the wet ingredients into the dry and stir to form a dough; this could take up to 5 minutes. It should be thick and easy to pick up and roll into a ball.

4   Roll between 2 sheets of nonstick baking paper to about 3mm (⅛ inch) thick. You can also achieve this by hand by just pressing the mix down between 2 sheets of nonstick baking paper, and smoothing it out. You need it to fit on your largest baking sheet.

5   Carefully peel off the top layer of paper, gently score out rectangular crackers and carefully move them, still on the baking paper to the large baking sheet.

6   Bake in the oven for 45 minutes until firm and golden. Every oven is different, so check them every 10 minutes. It might be they only need 35 minutes in your oven.

7   Once firm and golden, remove from the oven and place the baking sheet on a wire rack to cool. As soon as the sheet of crackers is cool enough to handle, flip them over and carefully peel off the baking paper, then leave on the wire rack until fully cold. Once cold, break them up into crackers. You can freeze them, or pop them in an airtight container and keep for up to 10 days at room temperature.

BAKES

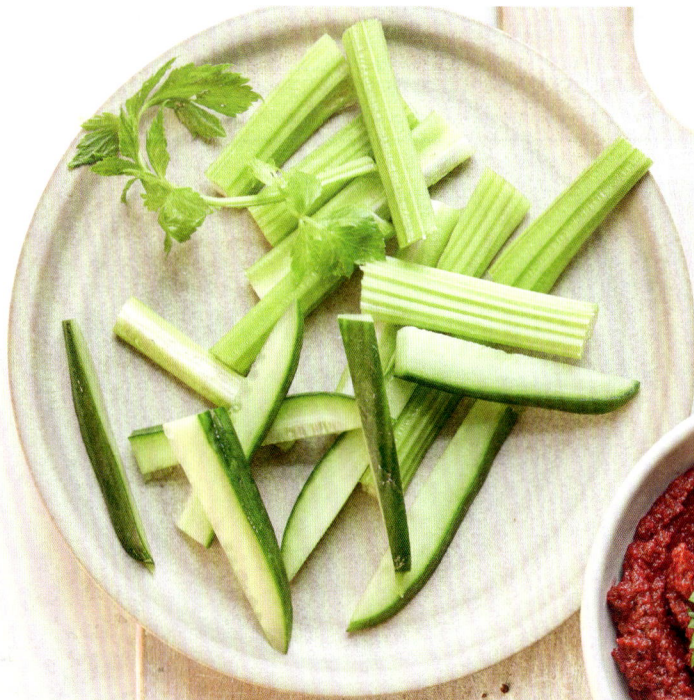

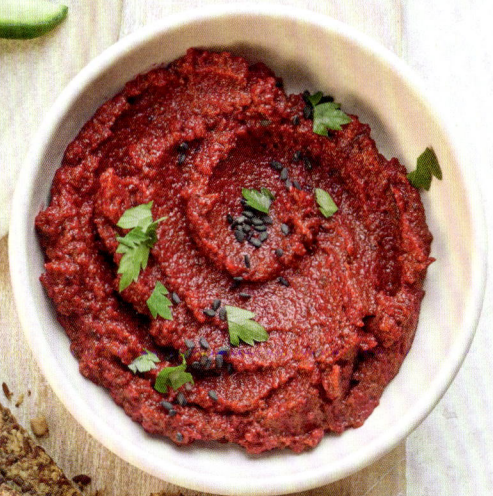

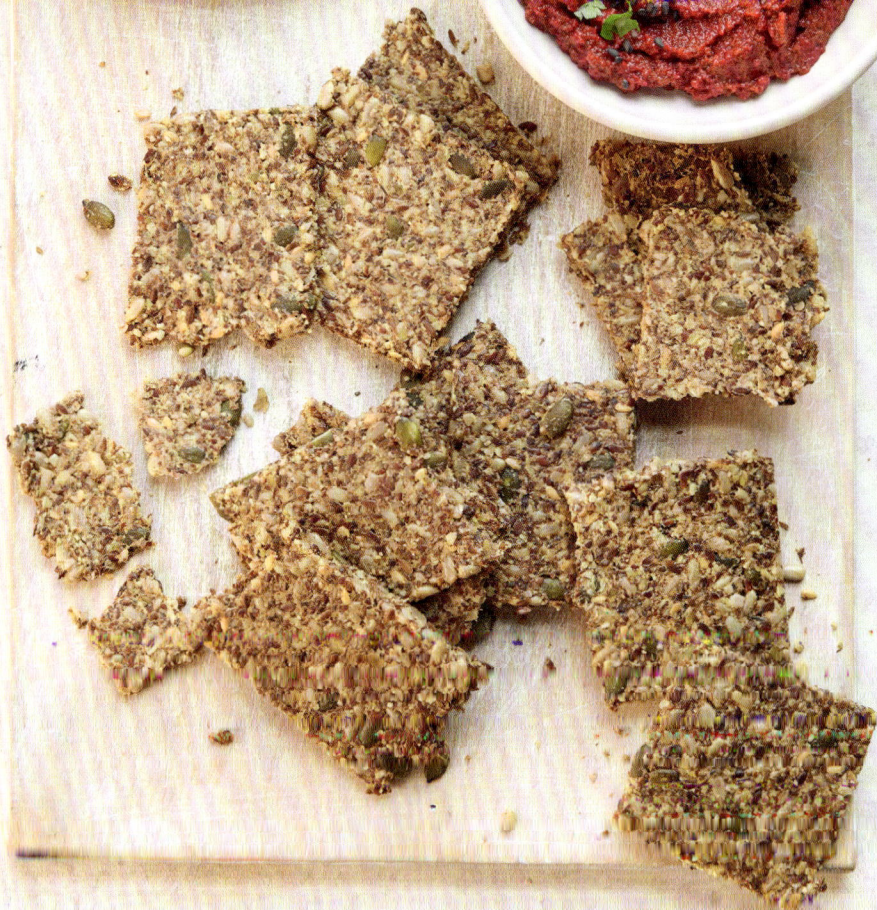

Occasional sweets

By their very nature, sweet treats and desserts are higher in calories. However, the ingredients used in the recipes here are certainly more health-friendly than usual. You will see that the carbs numbers contained in the recipes are low, which will benefit those living with diabetes, and there is a large and varied selection to keep you inspired! Sweet treats have their place in our lives as an occasional treat, but remember your main goal is avoiding weight regain.

As you will see, some of the recipes here are much lighter in calories than others. Where recipes use butter and nuts they will be more calorific, so please do save these for special occasions or when you have lots of mouths to feed, and importantly when you can join in too! There's nothing worse than making a cake to share with a friend, only for them to leave you with 10 slices still to eat...

Greek yogurt: a best friend for the sweet-toothed

Greek yogurt not only contains protein and fats, but it is also full of gut-friendly bacteria. Perhaps that fact is not top of your priority list when you're ransacking the cupboard for a sweet fix, but looking after our gut microbiome is something we should all be doing.

Someone once said to me that a dessert just has to have 'dessertness' (disclaimer: it's not a real word). I think he could read my puzzled face, as he added, 'You know, it has to have one or all of those characteristics that we love: a creaminess, a tanginess, a richness to it.' I got it! If it has indulgence to it, it has dessertness.

This leads me back to Greek yogurt. Greek yogurt has dessertness. It is the perfect base for creating lower-calorie and low-carb desserts to satisfy anyone's sweet tooth, because it is creamy, tangy and rich. Turning Greek yogurt into something indulgent and dessert-like, while keeping it low-calorie, is easier than you might think. You can pop it in a nice little serving dish and add sprinkles of dark chocolate, raspberries and a small drizzle of nut butter... and you have effortlessly created something with dessertness. Get creative and experiment with different flavours and toppings to find your perfect combination.

Here's how Greek yogurt ticks the dessertness box:

It is luxuriously thick and **CREAMY** in texture and feels indulgent on its own

The **TANGINESS** of Greek yogurt adds depth and complexity to desserts, balancing out sweetness

It is **VERSATILE**. It can be easily flavoured and paired with toppings and mix-ins to create endless possibilities

OCCASIONAL SWEETS

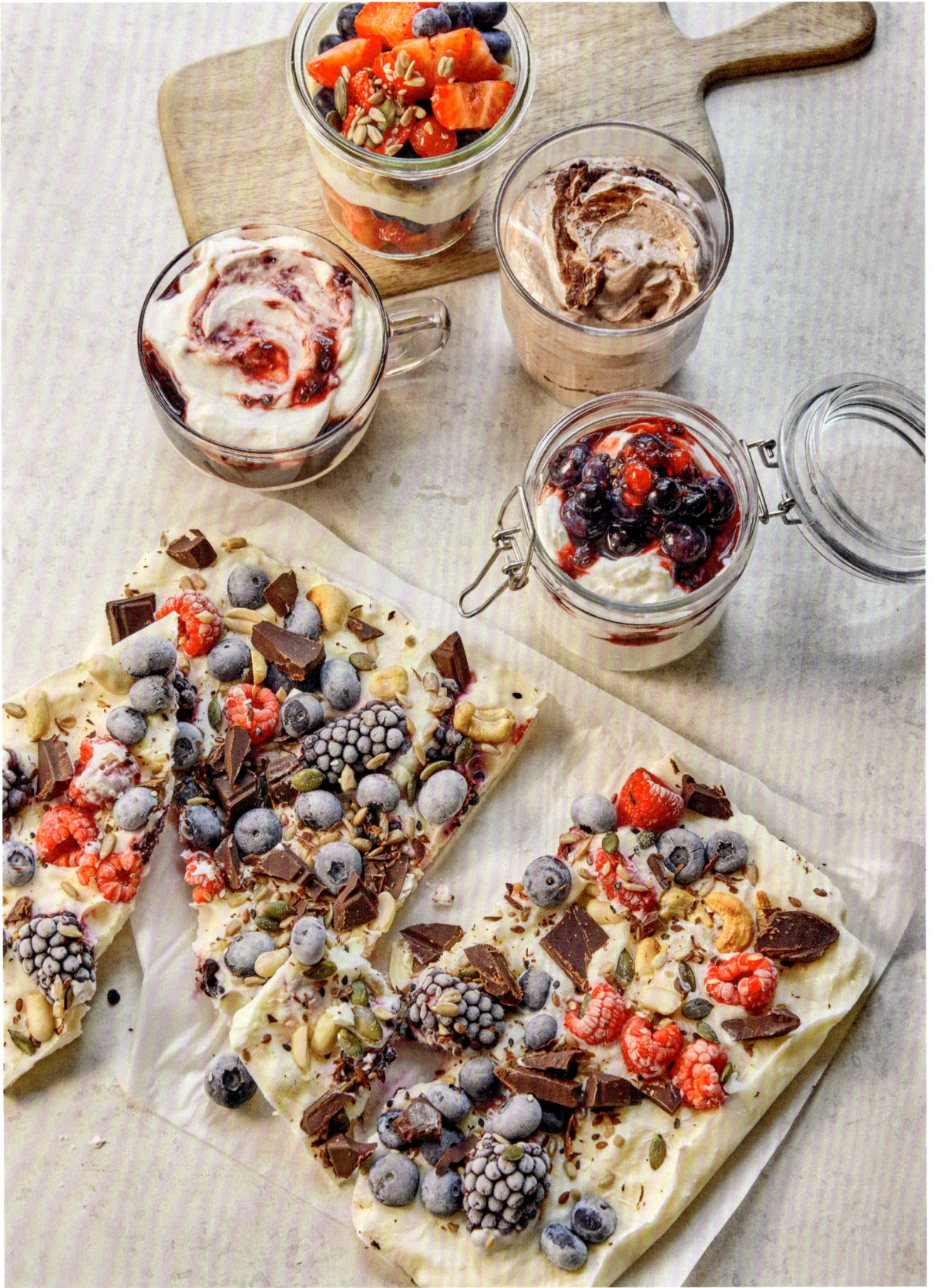

HOW TO ELEVATE GREEK YOGURT INTO A DESSERT DREAM

FRUIT COMPOTE

Simmer fresh or frozen berries in a pan, breaking them down with a wooden spoon to release their juices. Once thickened, add a little sweetener (such as erythritol). Spoon the warm compote over a small pot of chilled Greek yogurt to create a fruity, indulgent treat that mixes warm with cool.

CHOCOLATE-GREEK YOGURT MOUSSE

Mix Greek yogurt with unsweetened cocoa powder, a splash of sugar-free vanilla extract and 1 teaspoon powdered sweetener. Whisk together until smooth and airy, then chill to create a velvety chocolate mousse-like dessert.

FROZEN YOGURT BARK

Spread Greek yogurt on to a baking sheet or silicone mat (I find silicone works best) and sprinkle with toppings such as berries, seeds and finely chopped dark chocolate. Freeze until firm, then break into bark-like pieces for a satisfying and crunchy dessert.

FRUIT AND NUT PARFAIT

Spoon Greek yogurt into a jar, then add a layer of chopped nuts and seeds and a sweet fruit such as chopped mango. Repeat with Greek yogurt, nuts and seeds and fruit to make a layered dessert.

BLACKBERRY JAM YOGURT POTS

Spoon 1 tablespoon of my Low-Sugar Blackberry Jam (see page 184) in a small jar, followed by a layer of 40g (1½oz) Greek yogurt. Add another tablespoon of jam and finish off with another 40g (1½oz) layer of Greek yogurt. Chill before serving.

OCCASIONAL SWEETS

LOW-SUGAR BLACKBERRY JAM

MAKES
1 JAR

PREP TIME
LESS THAN 5 MINS

COOK TIME
15 MINS

300g (10½oz) blackberries

3 tablespoons powdered sweetener, plus more if needed

2 teaspoons xanthan gum, or chia seeds

PER JAR	
NET CARBS	17G
FIBRE	15G
PROTEIN	3.9G
FAT	0.6G
KCAL	132

Once you start to really consider what you are putting into your body, you'll want to investigate the ingredients listed on product packaging. One of those with the most power to shock is jam. Sugar is often the first ingredient listed, meaning it is the main ingredient, often to camouflage lower-quality fruit and / or to extend shelf life. Knowledge is power: we can vote with our wallets and stop purchasing ultra-processed foods that will have a negative impact on our blood sugars.

It is important to beware of what is called the 'health halo' effect: don't be fooled by labels screaming 'sugar-free' or 'all natural'. Always read the packaging, because often the ingredients will be anything but natural. In this way, you'll reduce the possibility of consuming hidden sugars and additives. Homemade jam will be far healthier for you, can be adjusted to your taste and your blood sugars will thank you for it. When making jam yourself, ideally opt for berries, as they are high in fibre and more gentle on blood glucose levels due to their low carb count. As these jams do not contain any preservatives, please note that their shelf life, when kept in the refrigerator, is about 10 days.

1 Tip the blackberries into a small saucepan over a high heat. Press down on the berries to release their juice. Once they start to sizzle, reduce the heat, but keep pressing them down to release the juice. You should have a decent amount of liquid now, so cook it for about 10 minutes to reduce it down.

2 Once it has thickened a little, add the sweetener and xanthan gum or chia. Now press the blackberries through a sieve into a bowl. You will have to persevere with this until you have separated all the seeds from the jam.

3 Once you have deseeded as much as possible, taste the mixture and see if you want to stir in a little more sweetener. Spoon the mixture into a jar, seal, cool and keep in the refrigerator until required.

Chocolate

Oh, my favourite ingredient! When I was young, I dreamed of one day having a swimming pool filled with chocolate, and of being a chocolatier, too. Granted, I didn't have diabetes back then! I am yet to achieve either of those goals… but never say never. However, I have learned how to make some pretty spectacular chocolate desserts over the years.

Chocolate is high in calories primarily due to its fat content, especially milk chocolate, which has more sugar. However, dark chocolate (70 per cent cocoa solids and higher) has little added sugar and is much lower in carbohydrates. This makes it a more sensible option for those living with diabetes, as it has less impact on blood sugar levels.

There are two ways to melt chocolate safely:

Bain-marie method

Place broken-up or chopped chocolate in a heatproof (glass or metal) bowl set over a pan of simmering water. The base of the bowl should not touch the water. The steam from the simmering water will gently heat the bowl and melt the chocolate without burning it. This method allows for precise control over the melting process and prevents the chocolate from overheating.

Microwave method

Place broken-up or chopped chocolate into a microwave-proof bowl and heat it at short intervals, typically of 15–30 seconds, stirring between each interval. This is quicker, but it requires careful attention to prevent the chocolate from burning or overheating, which can cause it to seize (clump up) or become grainy.

2-INGREDIENT CHOCOLATE MOUSSE

SERVES
8

400ml (14fl oz) can of coconut milk (see below)

120g (4¼oz) chocolate (70 per cent cocoa solids), melted (see page 185)

To serve (optional)

chocolate shavings (70 per cent cocoa solids)

raspberries

PER SERVING	
NET CARBS	6.4G
FIBRE	1.8G
PROTEIN	2G
FAT	15G
KCAL	170

PREP TIME
10 MINS, PLUS CHILLING TIME

By using just two simple storecupboard ingredients, you can create a very decadent dessert. This recipe has been tried and enjoyed by thousands of people across the world, at wellness retreats, events, cooking classes and charity events for people living with diabetes. The incredible feedback I've received means it just has to go into this book for you, too. It is a firm favourite in many households and a game-changer for those living with diabetes looking for a simple, no-frills pudding that tastes good and is lower in calories and carbs. You can prep it ahead, too.

If you would like to use a chocolate with a higher percentage of cocoa, please do so, but be mindful that it will reduce the overall net carbs.

1 Pour the coconut milk into a heatproof bowl and whisk for 30 seconds to get lots of air into it.

2 Carefully pour the melted chocolate into the coconut milk, whisking all the time.

3 Continue to whisk until combined: the more you whisk, the better the mousse will be.

4 Pour into ramekins. Decorate with shaved dark chocolate or 1–2 raspberries, if you like. Place in the refrigerator for at least 3 hours until set.

RECIPE TIP

Brands of coconut milk may vary – some are more watery than others which could prevent it from firming up, so to avoid this I recommend a brand with a coconut extract of at least 55 per cent. Check the labels for minimal ingredients – preferably with just coconut and water, and avoid those with emulsifiers and additives if possible.

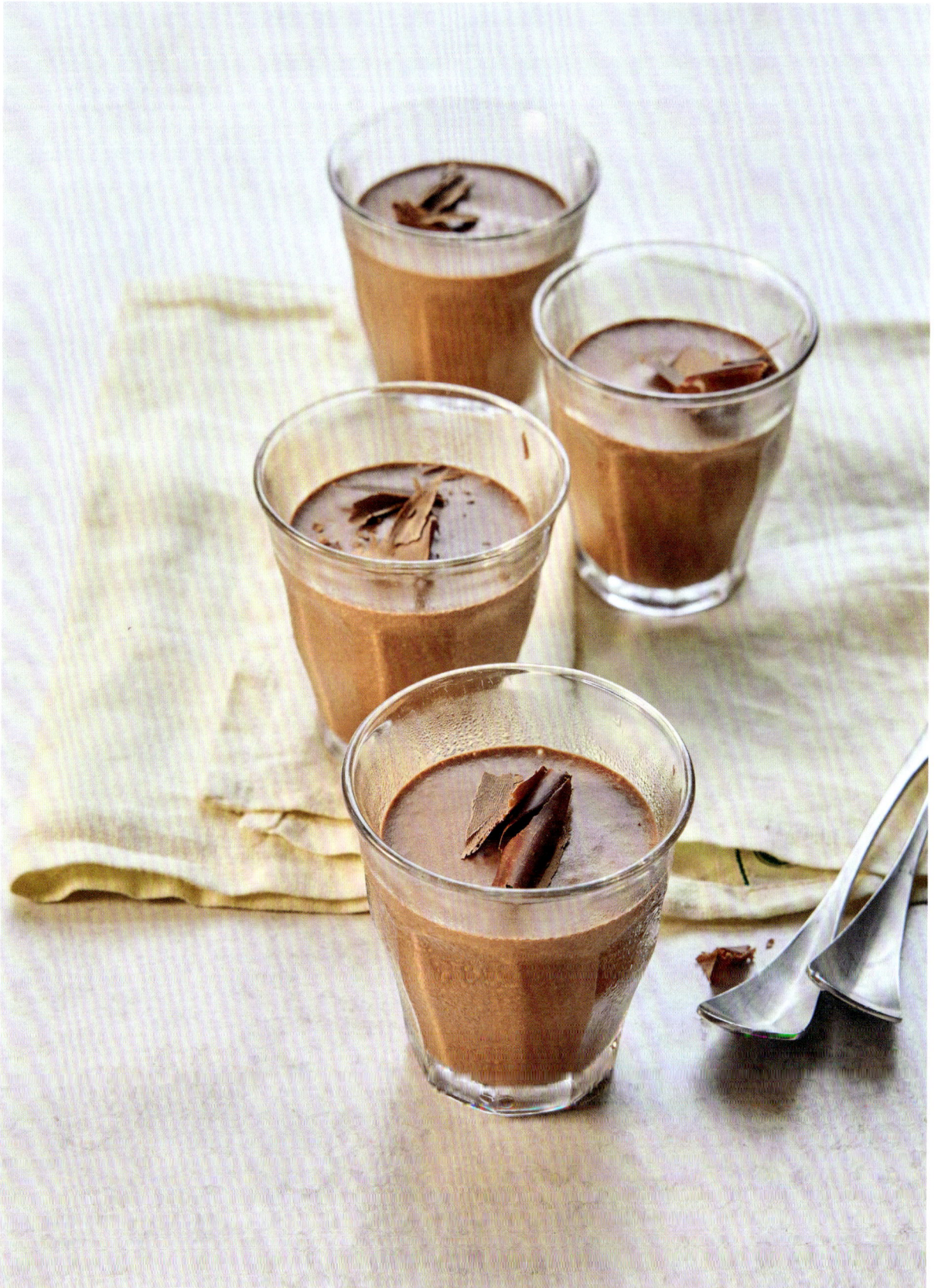

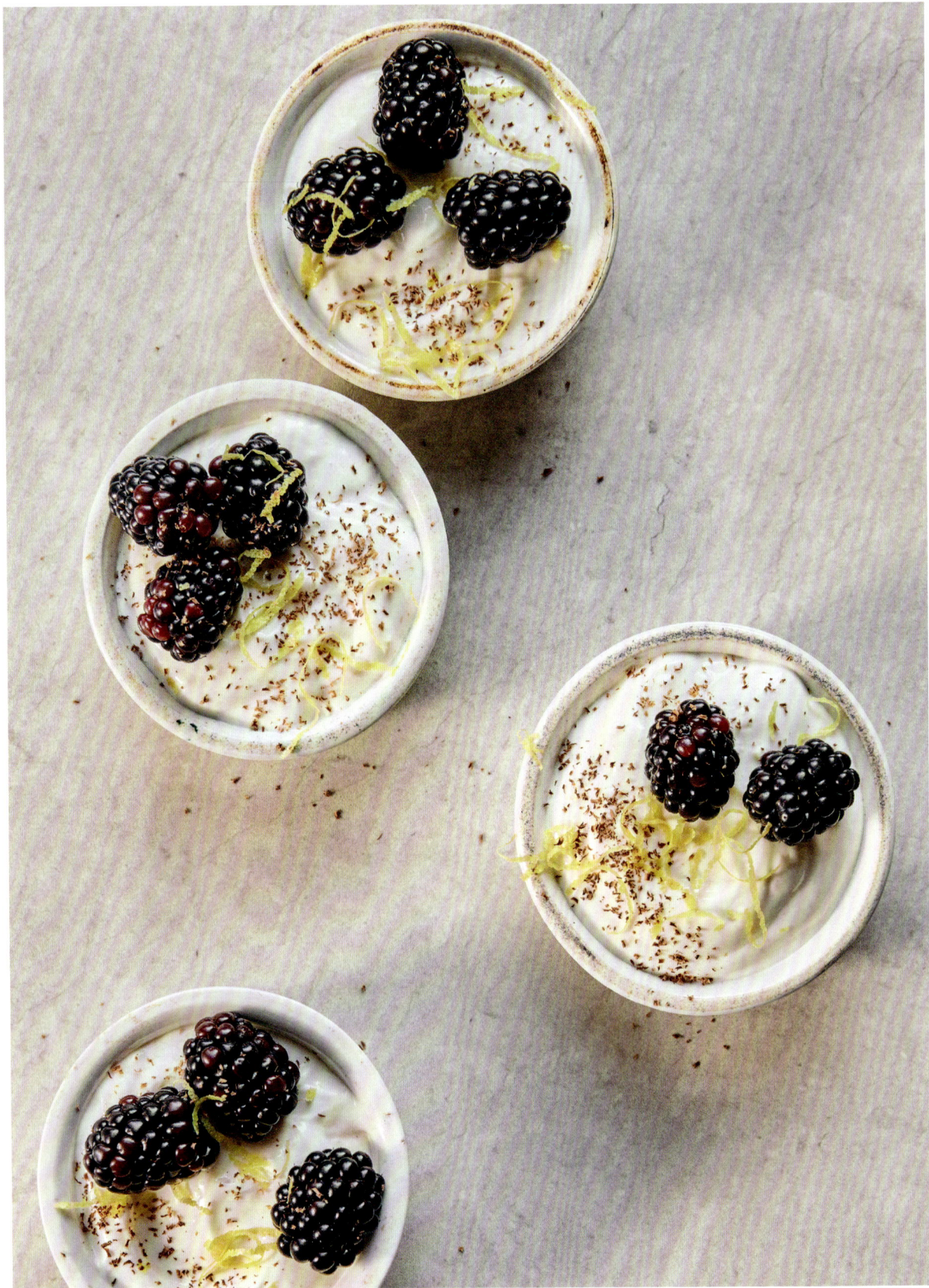

CREAMY NO-BAKE LEMON CHEESECAKE POTS

SERVES
4

PREP TIME
10 MINS, PLUS CHILLING TIME

COOK TIME
5 MINS

200g (7oz) cream cheese (reduced fat, if you like)

100g (3½oz) Greek yogurt

finely grated zest and juice of 1 lemon

2–3 tablespoons powdered sweetener, such as erythritol or stevia, to taste

1 teaspoon sugar-free vanilla extract

1 tablespoonpowdered gelatine

4 tablespoons boiling water

To serve (optional)

1 teaspoon chopped chocolate (70 per cent cocoa solids)

a few fresh berries

These no-bake, base-free lemon cheesecake pots are so quick to make, and they're creamy, tangy, sweet and satisfying. Perfect for an after-dinner treat to share. Powdered sweetener works best in recipes such as this, where no heat is used.

1 In a mixing bowl, combine the cream cheese, yogurt, lemon zest and juice, powdered sweetener and vanilla extract. Mix until smooth and well combined.

2 In a small bowl, sprinkle the gelatine powder over the measured boiling water and stir until completely dissolved. Allow to cool slightly.

3 Pour the slightly cooled gelatine mixture into the cream cheese mixture. Mix until fully incorporated.

4 Divide the mixture evenly between 4 small pots or ramekins. Cover and put in the refrigerator for 2–3 hours, or until set.

5 Once set, decorate with chopped chocolate or fresh berries and serve.

PER SERVING	
NET CARBS	2.6G (3.7G)
FIBRE	0G
PROTEIN	7.4G (9.3G)
FAT	18G (5.5G)
KCAL	207 (104)

RECIPE TIP

The nutritional information (see box) has been calculated using full-fat cream cheese and Greek yogurt, with figures for the low-fat cream cheese and fat-free Greek yogurt in brackets. If you use low-fat or fat-free versions, please be mindful that this will significantly change the information (specifically calories, which will decrease, and carbs, which might increase a little). I tend to use full-fat ingredients for the Step 3 recipes in this book, as these will nourish you and keep you satiated. If you are using low-fat alternatives, seek out products that only use single ingredients, with no added sweeteners or sugars.

CHOCOLATE TORTE

MAKES
10 SLICES

PREP TIME
10 MINS, PLUS CHILLING

COOK TIME
20 MINS

butter, for the tin

550g (1lb 4oz) sweet potato, peeled and chopped into cubes

160g (5¾oz) chocolate (70 per cent cocoa solids), chopped

seasonal berries, to serve

For the icing

60g (2¼oz) chocolate (70 per cent cocoa solids)

30ml (2 tablespoons) milk (I used unsweetened almond milk)

PER SLICE	
NET CARBS	18G
FIBRE	3.8G
PROTEIN	2.7G
FAT	9.5G
KCAL	175

A simple, scrumptious, fudgy and flourless no-bake chocolate torte. This pudding needs no more words.

1 Butter a 20cm (8 inch) cake tin with a removeable base, and line with nonstick baking paper.

2 Place the sweet potato in a saucepan of boiling water, cover and simmer for about 15 minutes until soft. Drain, then tip the sweet potato straight into a blender. Add the chopped chocolate to the blender: it will start melting into the sweet potato. Blend until you have created a smooth batter. You will have to scrape down the sides a couple of times to fully mix all of the ingredients.

3 Pour the mixture into the prepared tin and refrigerate for about 5 hours until set.

4 Once set, you can make the icing. Melt the chocolate (see page 185 for the methods). Once melted, add the almond milk little by little, whisking, until glossy. Pour over the torte and tip from side to side until evenly coated, then return to the refrigerator until firm. (This will keep chilled for up to 4 days.)

5 Carefully remove the torte from the tin and serve with seasonal berries.

RECIPE TIP

If you have left your sweet potato in the blender for a while and it has cooled too much to melt the chocolate, then melt the chocolate separately (see page 185 for the methods) before adding it to the sweet potato and blending.

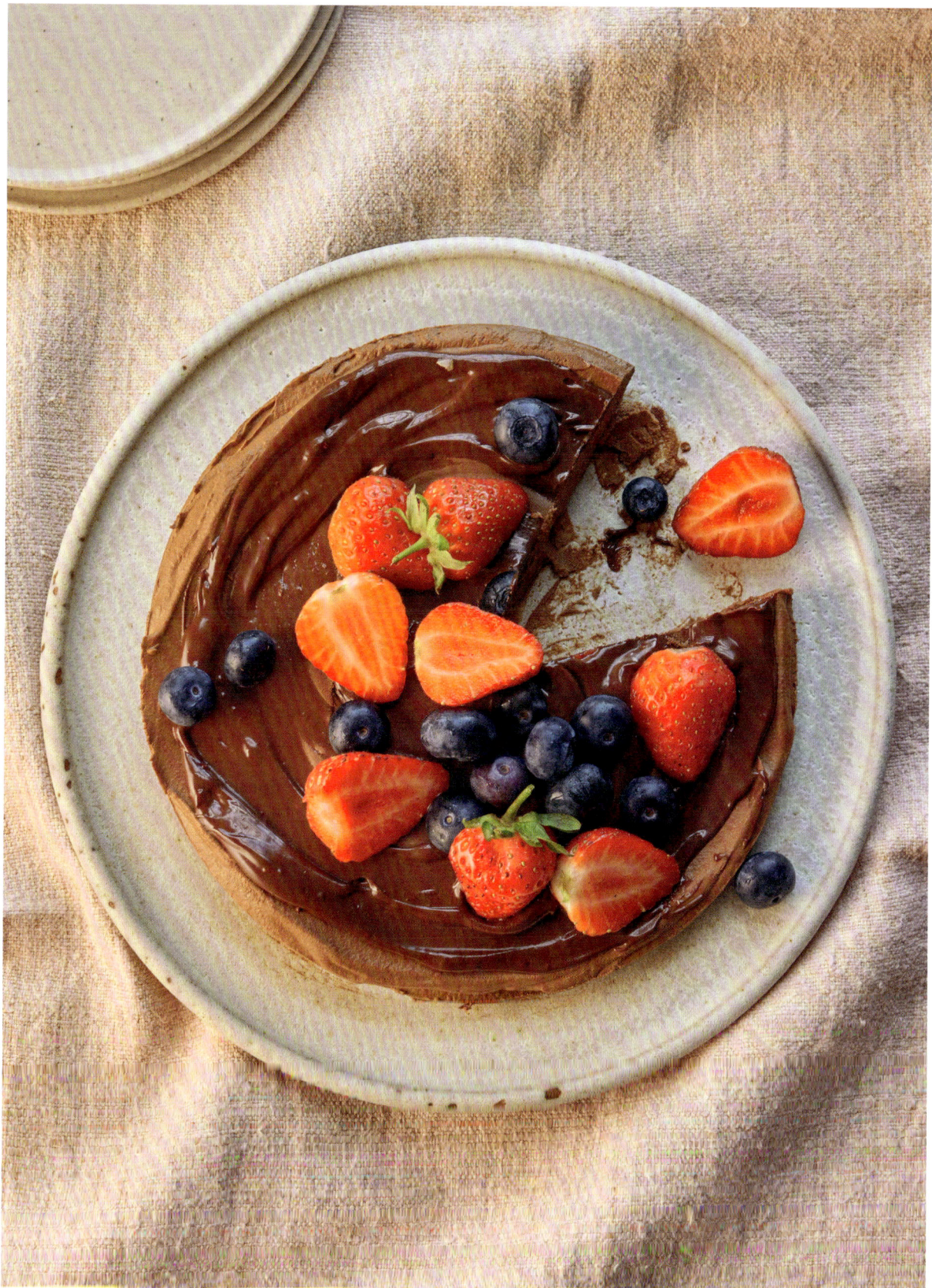

FLOURLESS CHOCOLATE SPONGE
WITH SWEET MASCARPONE CREAM

MAKES
12 SQUARES

PREP TIME
20 MINS

COOK TIME
25 MINS

For the sponge

flavourless oil, for the tin

125g (4½oz) Greek yogurt (I use additive-free, fat-free)

50g (1¾oz) brown granulated sweetener (I use erythritol)

2 large eggs

2 tablespoons milk (I used unsweetened almond milk)

50g (1¾oz) ground flaxseeds / linseeds, or ground almonds

20g (¾oz) coconut flour or gluten-free plain flour

20g (¾oz) cocoa powder

1 teaspoon baking powder

For the cream

120g (4¼oz) mascarpone cheese

¼ teaspoon pure vanilla bean paste, or 1 teaspoon sugar-free vanilla extract

10g (¼oz) powdered sweetener

To serve (optional)

grated chocolate (70 per cent cocoa solids)

sugar-free sprinkles

Sometimes when you reduce your carb intake, you might see a spike in fat consumption and therefore calories, however, not with this recipe – no one will be able to tell how low in carbs and added sugars this is. You can bake the sponge in advance and freeze it in individual portions. It can then be defrosted and the mascarpone cream added when you're ready to serve (mix it up proportionately, according to the number of portions you want to serve). You will need a 900g (2lb) loaf tin, or a square cake tin of equivalent volume.

1   Preheat the oven to 180°C (350°F), Gas Mark 4. Lightly oil a 900g (2lb) loaf tin and line it with nonstick baking paper.

2   Place the Greek yogurt and granulated sweetener in a food processor. Add the eggs and milk and beat until thoroughly mixed. (Or beat by hand in a bowl with a wooden spoon.)

3   Add the ground flaxseeds or almonds, the coconut flour, cocoa powder and baking powder and mix until the cake batter is well-combined.

4   Bake for up to 25 minutes until a knife or skewer can be inserted into the middle and be withdrawn completely clean. Transfer to a wire rack to cool.

5   Pop the mascarpone, vanilla and powdered sweetener into a bowl and mix. Once the cake is fully cooled, use a spoon to dollop the cream on to the cake and carefully spread it out.

6   Decorate with grated chocolate or sugar-free sprinkles, if you like.

PER SQUARE	
NET CARBS	1.3G
FIBRE	2.3G
PROTEIN	4G
FAT	7.8G
KCAL	96

RECIPE TIP

I use granulated erythritol for baking and powdered erythritol for the mascarpone cream, but feel free to use your preferred alternative. However, be aware that some sweeteners can produce a very pungent aftertaste, so err on the side of caution and start by using a small amount and add more until you reach the required level of sweetness.

BERRY AND NUT CHOCOLATE BARK

MAKES
22 PIECES

PREP TIME
10 MINS

COOK TIME
5 MINS

250g (9oz) chocolate (70 per cent cocoa solids)

100g (3½oz) mixed nuts, chopped

200g (7oz) strawberries, hulled and sliced

sea salt flakes

PER PIECE	
NET CARBS	4.7G
FIBRE	2G
PROTEIN	2.3G
FAT	7.1G
KCAL	97

The perfect chocolate boost to keep in the freezer, ready to be grabbed and eaten in those moments where you feel the need for a treat. As it is frozen, it will take time to make, appreciate and savour. If you do not like strawberries, use any other berry you prefer. Berries are the best choice, as they work well with chocolate and are low in carbs, so they make a good choice for those with diabetes.

1   Line a large freezerproof baking dish with nonstick baking paper.

2   Melt the chocolate (see page 185 for the methods).

3   Add three-quarters of the nuts to the chocolate and stir through until fully coated.

4   Spread the strawberries evenly over the prepared baking dish. Pour the chocolate over the strawberries until they are all coated in chocolate. Sprinkle the remaining nuts on top and sprinkle with sea salt flakes.

5   Place in the freezer and freeze until set. Carefully cut into 22 squares using a hot knife (see below), then store in an airtight container in the freezer.

RECIPE TIP   The easiest way to cut chocolate is with a hot knife, and this also applies to chocolate bark. Run the blade of a sharp knife under boiling water (from a kettle), then carefully slice the chocolate. You might need to pour the boiling water over the blade a few times during the chopping process.

COURGETTE AND OLIVE OIL CAKE
WITH LEMON ICING

OCCASIONAL SWEETS

SERVES
10 SLICES

PREP TIME
20 MIN

COOK TIME
35–40 MINS

For the cake

unsalted butter, for the tin

3 large eggs

30ml light olive oil

200g (7oz) Greek yogurt

1 teaspoon sugar-free vanilla extract

15g (½oz) granulated sweetener

135g (4¾oz) ground almonds

10g (¼oz) coconut flour or gluten-free plain flour

100g (3½oz) courgette, grated

For the icing

3 tablespoons icing sugar (alternatively use powdered sweetener icing sugar)

2 tablespoons lemon juice

1 teaspoon finely grated lemon zest, plus more to serve

1 tablespoon arrowroot

PER SLICE	
NET CARBS	6.3G
FIBRE	1.8G
PROTEIN	6.6G
FAT	14G
KCAL	185

A cake which also works well as a pudding. You may well find you're on the receiving end of a sharp look of alarm when you tell people the surprise ingredient... but please do not let this wonderful vegetable put you off. The courgette adds a delicious amount of moisture and is vital in this recipe. The cake is great sliced up and served with an extra dollop of Greek yogurt.

You only need a little grated lemon zest, so freeze the rest in a little pot for another time.

1 Preheat the oven to 180°C (350°F), Gas Mark 4. Lightly butter a 900g (2lb) loaf tin and line with nonstick baking paper.

2 Place the eggs in a mixing bowl and whisk them until pale and frothy. Whisk in the olive oil, Greek yogurt and vanilla. Continue to whisk: you want to create a custard.

3 Add the sweetener, ground almonds and coconut flour. Using a wooden spoon, stir until you have a smooth batter. Fold in the grated courgette and stir until combined.

4 Pour the batter into the prepared tin. Bake for 35–40 minutes or until a knife or skewer can be inserted into the middle and be withdrawn completely clean. Transfer to a wire rack to cool.

5 Place all the ingredients for the lemon icing in a small mixing bowl and stir together. If you need more liquid, then add a little cold water, but only 1 tablespoon at a time. The icing needs to be of a pourable consistency.

6 When the cake is cold, pour on the icing and spread it evenly over the cake with a spatula. Scatter lemon zest on top and leave to set.

7 Remove from the loaf tin and serve.

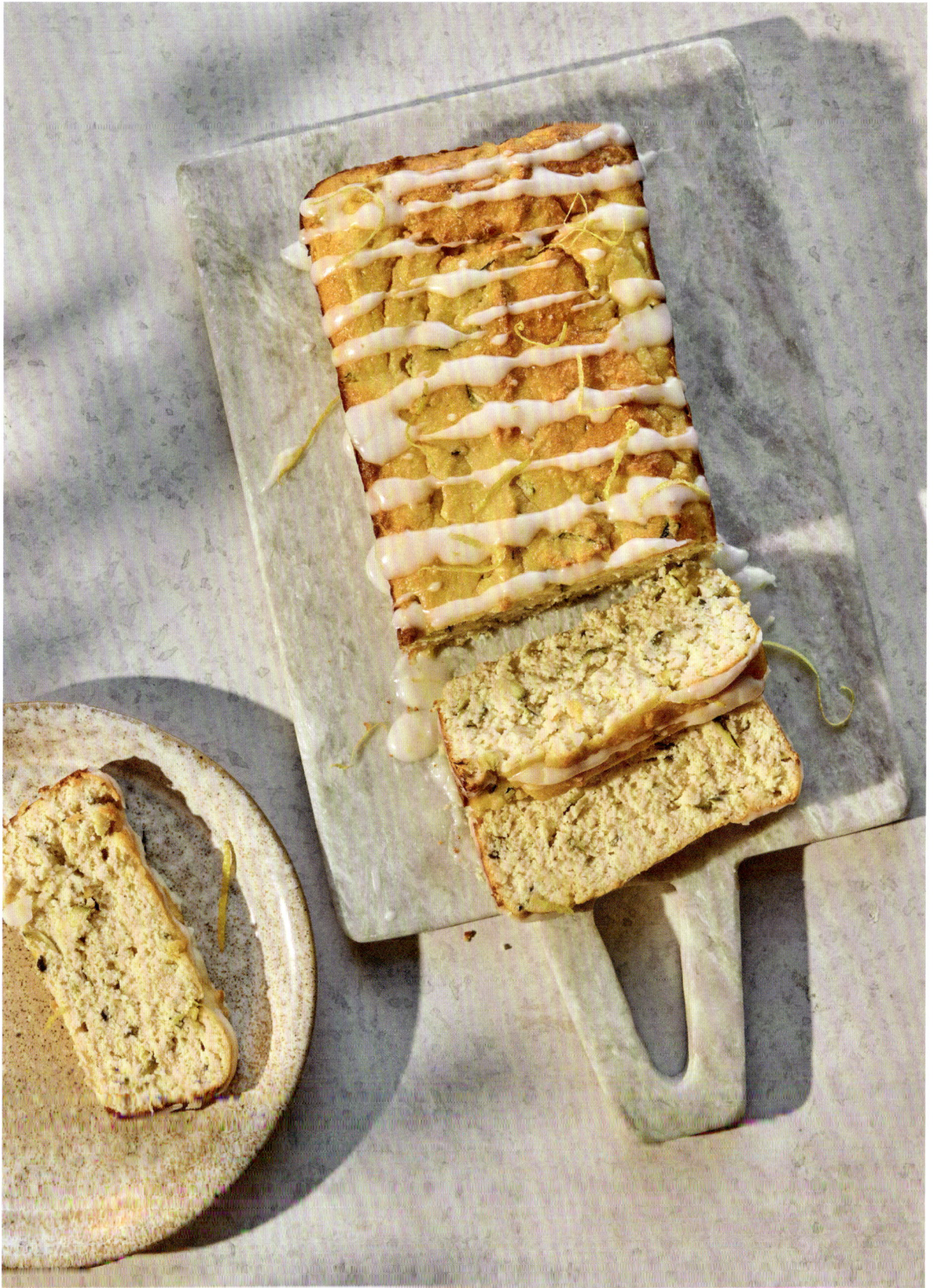

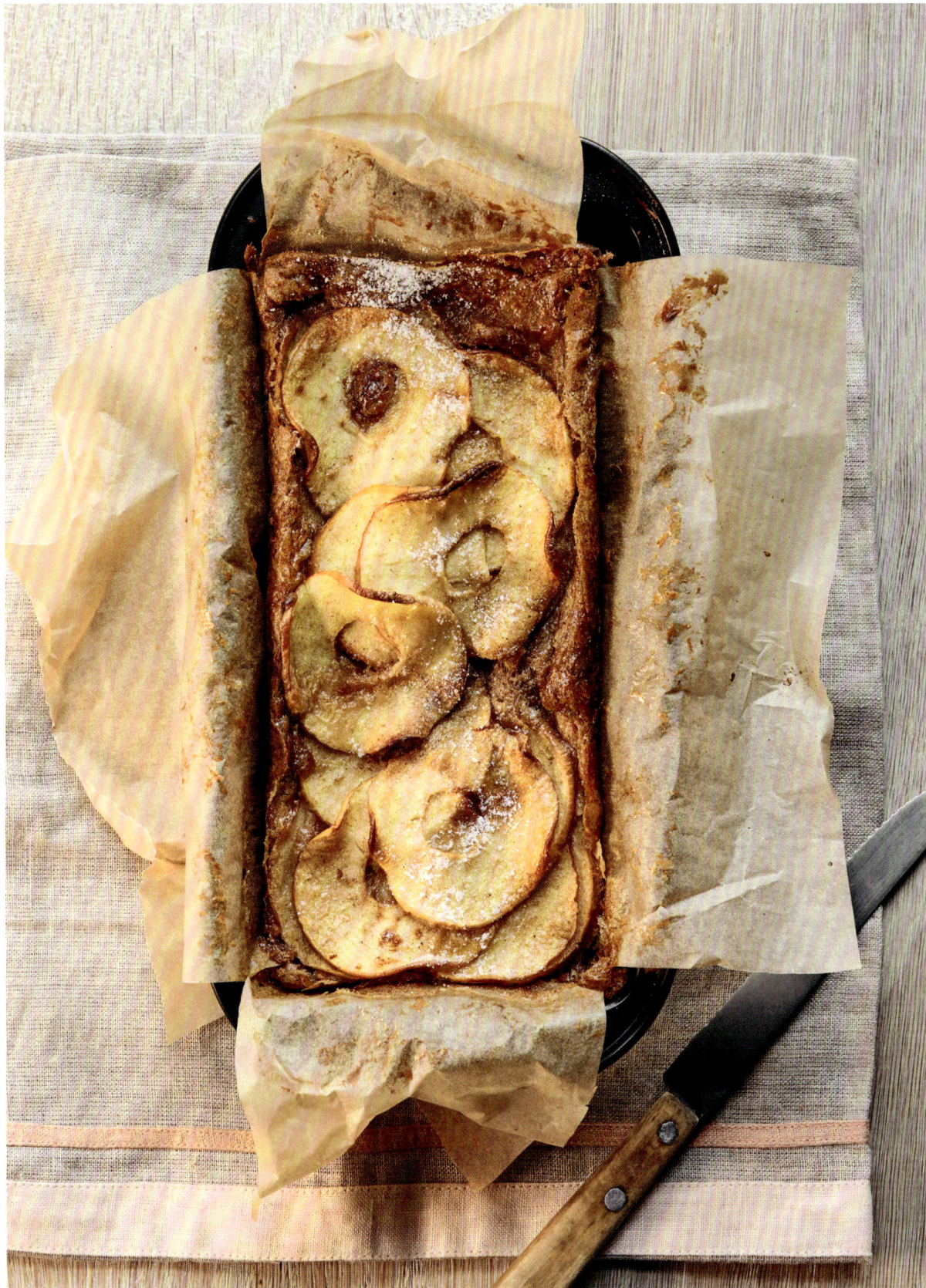

APPLE LAYERED CAKE

SERVES
6

PREP TIME
15 MINS

COOK TIME
50 MINS

2 large eggs

40g (1½oz) granulated sweetener, plus more to dust

2 teaspoons ground cinnamon

40ml (3 tablespoons) unsweetened almond milk

2 teaspoons sugar-free vanilla extract

30g (1oz) unsalted butter, melted, plus extra to butter the tin

20g (¾oz) arrowroot

pinch of sea salt

2 teaspoons baking powder

450g (1lb) large apples (about 4)

PER SLICE	
NET CARBS	13G
FIBRE	1.3G
PROTEIN	3.2G
FAT	6.4G
KCAL	125

When we bought our home, my husband presented me with an apple tree. We were very excited to plant it in what was, at the time, a big rectangular mud bath. Well, seven years in and the apple tree, though a little thicker in trunk, is still only 1 metre (3ft) tall, but it does yield a once-a-year crop of wonderful apples. During late summer, my daughters pick the apples and we make a whole host of delectable recipes, including this thick, dense and sweet cake. It is healthier and contains less sugar than the traditional apple tart my mother used to make, but hopefully still memorably delicious!

1 Preheat the oven to 170°C (340°F), Gas Mark 3½. Butter a 900g (2lb) loaf tin and line the base with nonstick baking paper.

2 Place the eggs in a mixing bowl and whisk until frothy. Add the sweetener and cinnamon and continue to whisk until really fluffy and glossy. Add the almond milk, vanilla and melted butter and continue to whisk. Fold in the arrowroot, sea salt and baking powder and stir until combined.

3 Wash and core the apples. Then, using a mandolin or a very sharp knife, slice them finely and place in a bowl. If you like, halve the slices so they are crescent moon-shaped. You need to do this at the last minute, because the apple will brown very quickly once the flesh is exposed to air.

4 Add the apples to the batter and mix until coated.

5 Transfer to the prepared tin, sprinkle over a little granulated sweetener and bake for about 50 minutes until firm and golden brown.

6 Allow to cool before removing from the tin, slicing and serving. This will keep in the refrigerator for up to 3 days.

BERRY BOUNCY-CLOUD PUDDING

MAKES
8 SLICES

PREP TIME
15 MINS, PLUS RESTING TIME

COOK TIME
1½ HRS

4 large egg whites

20g (¾oz) granulated sweetener

15g (½oz) white caster sugar

2 teaspoons sugar-free vanilla extract

1 teaspoon apple cider vinegar

½ teaspoon cream of tartar

2 teaspoons arrowroot

For the topping

300g (10½oz) mixed frozen berries, defrosted

4 tablespoons powdered sweetener, plus extra to decorate

200g (7oz) fat-free extra-thick Greek yogurt

PER SLICE	
NET CARBS	6.2G
FIBRE	1G
PROTEIN	4.7G
FAT	0G
KCAL	47

A luscious, low-calorie pudding and an absolutely beautiful centrepiece, this resembles a pavlova with a soft, marshmallow consistency. My youngest daughter named it and the title couldn't be more perfect! I find a combination of sugar and sweetener works well for this recipe, but you can just use sweetener if you prefer.

1 Preheat the oven to 100°C (250°F), Gas Mark ½. Draw a 20cm (8 inch) diameter circle on a piece of nonstick baking paper and place it on a baking sheet.

2 Clean the bowl of a stand mixer or a mixing bowl and make sure it is completely dry. Using a stand mixer or hand whisk, whisk the egg whites into stiff peaks. Add the sweetener 1 tablespoon at a time, waiting 30 seconds between each addition. Once all the sweetener has been added, add the sugar and whisk for a further 30 seconds. Scrape down the sides of the bowl and mix for a further 3 minutes on medium-high until glossy. Add the vanilla extract, vinegar, cream of tartar and arrowroot. Mix for a final 2 minutes.

3 Spoon the mixture on to the prepared baking paper within the circle, smoothing it around.

4 Bake in the oven for 1½ hours, or until firm to the touch. Turn the oven off and leave the pavlova to cool with the door closed, then transfer to a cake stand or plate.

5 Tip the mixed berries into a bowl and stir in 2 tablespoons of the powdered sweetener. Stir the remaining sweetener into the Greek yogurt.

6 Top the pavlova with the yogurt mixture, berries and a sprinkle of extra powdered sweetener to decorate, then serve.

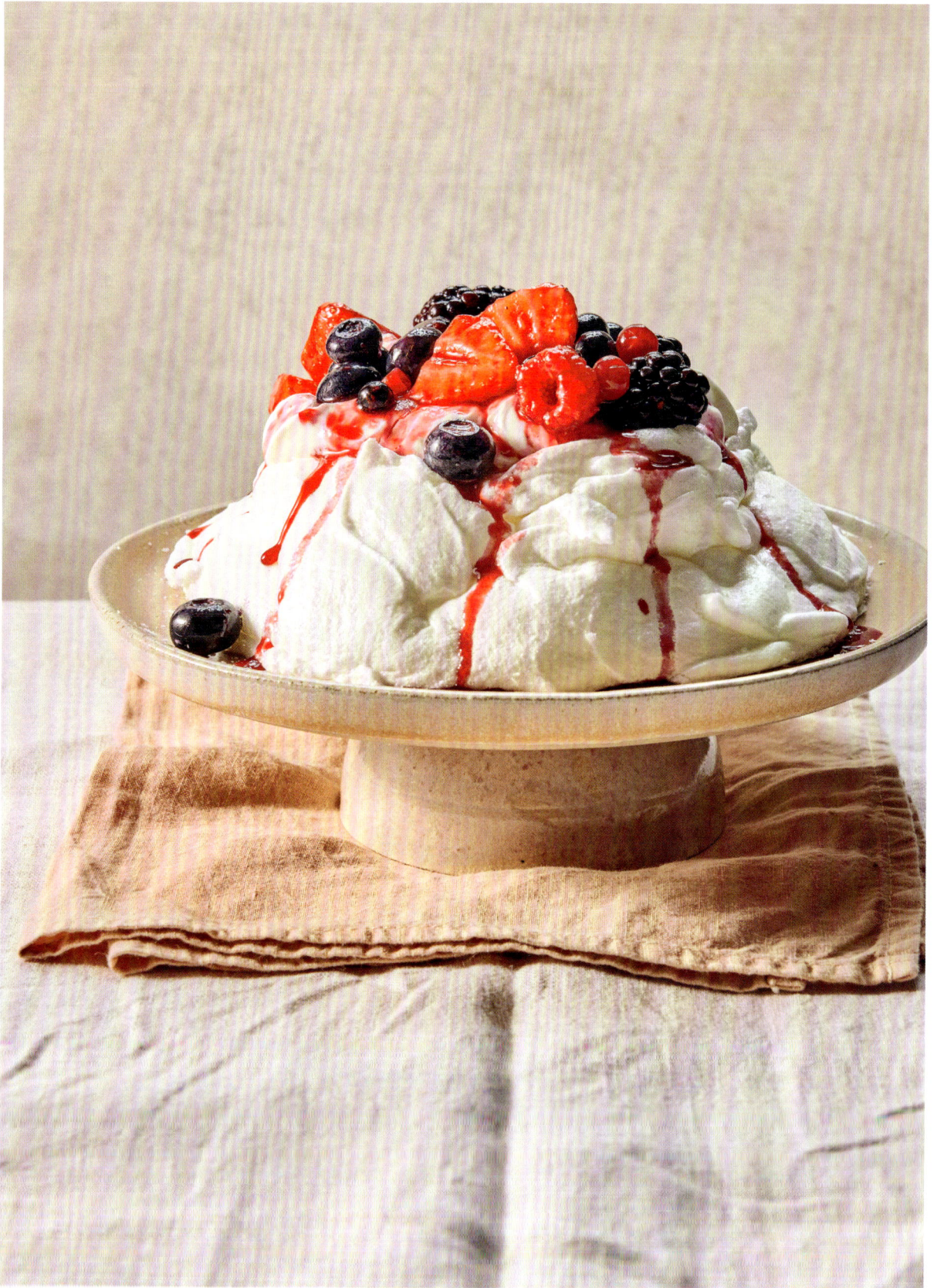

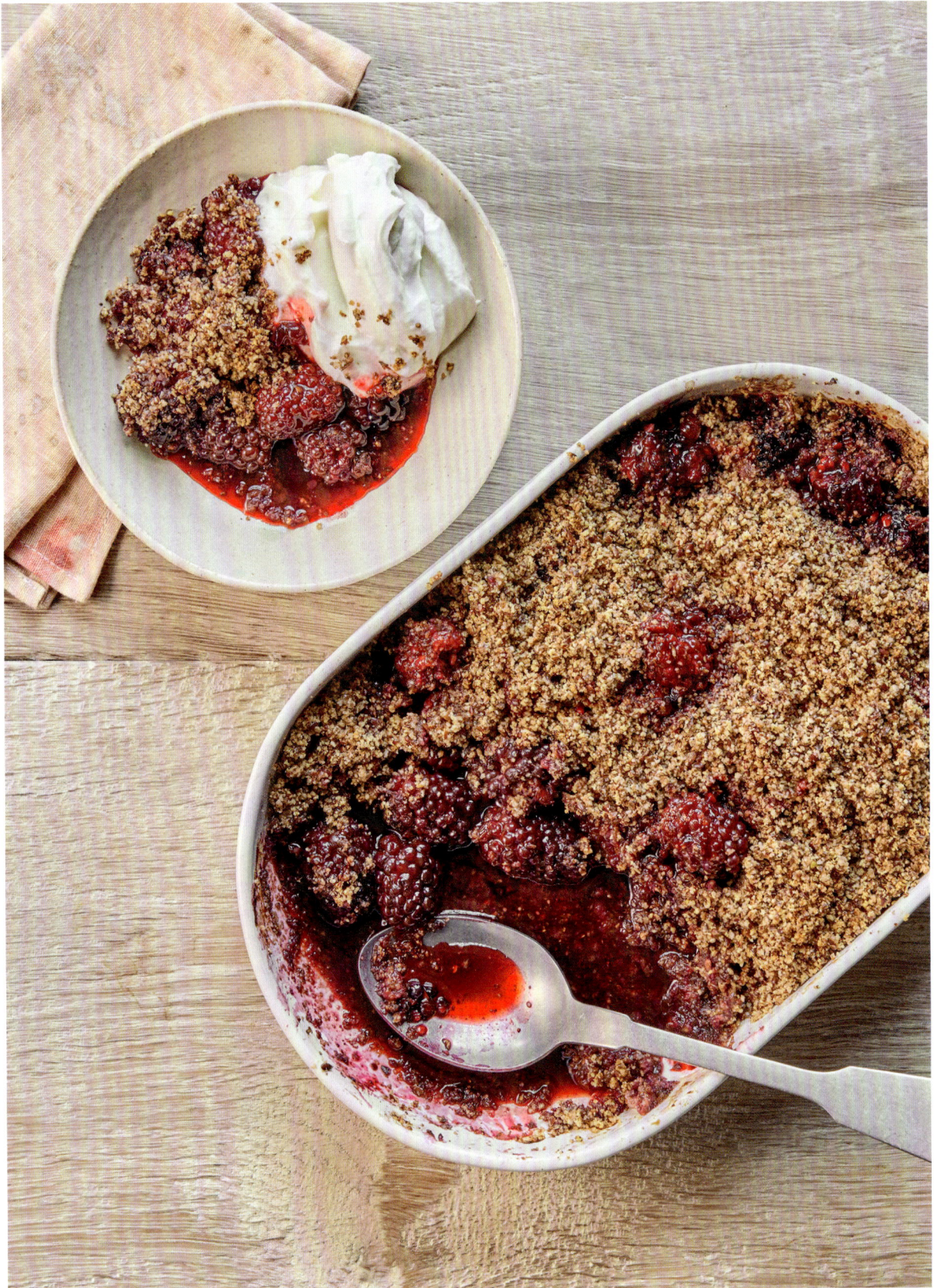

BLACKBERRY AND ALMOND CRUMBLE

SERVES
4

PREP TIME
10 MINS

COOK TIME
20 MINS

For the filling

400g (14oz) blackberries

2 tablespoons sweetener

For the topping

100g (3½oz) ground almonds,
   or any other milled nuts or seeds

100g (3½oz) ground flaxseed / linseed

2 tablespoons almond butter

40g (1½oz) unsalted butter,
   or coconut oil

1 teaspoon sweetener (optional)

1 teaspoon ground cinnamon
   (optional)

Greek yogurt or mascarpone cheese,
   to serve

PER SERVING	
NET CARBS	8G
FIBRE	14G
PROTEIN	11G
FAT	38G
KCAL	458

The best berries are free. In the UK, from August to October, the bushes are packed with blackberries and picking them is a great activity for the whole family, so grab containers and fill them up. Remove any stalks, then add the berries to a bowl with a mixture of 1 part vinegar to 3 parts water and leave to soak for 15 minutes. Drain in a colander, then dry them carefully, tip into freezer bags and freeze for use in the winter months. If you do not have access to blackberries, substitute with another berry of your choice. If buying pre-frozen, choose berries with a lower carb content (blackberries, strawberries, raspberries, redcurrants and blackcurrants) and avoid grapes which taste wonderfully sweet but will spike blood sugars.

1 Preheat the oven to 180°C (350°F), Gas Mark 4.

2 If the blackberries have been frozen, allow them to defrost, then place in a colander to drain off any excess liquid (this could be caught in a bowl and transferred to a bottle to use in cordial). Stir in the sweetener and place in a dish ready for baking. If the blackberries have not been frozen, place them into the dish with 50ml (1¾fl oz) boiling water along with the sweetener. Thoroughly mix everything together.

3 For the topping, place all the ingredients in a bowl and rub them together with your fingertips to form crumbs. Scatter the crumble mix on top of the fruit, covering it completely.

4 Bake for 20–25 minutes in the middle of the oven until the crumble is a light golden brown and the berries are bubbling through. Serve with some Greek yogurt or mascarpone.

MEAL PLANS

STEP 1

In Step 1, you will be consuming three smoothies, shakes or soups (see pages 34–54), plus a low-starch vegetable plate (see pages 56–71) per day, about 800 calories in total. The smoothies and shakes recipes in this book are single portions to ensure they are fresh and taste their best, and – importantly – that there is no room for overindulging. You can also continue to enjoy drinking tea or coffee with up to 100ml (3½oz) skimmed milk per day (47 calories, 3.6g protein), and no sugar.

MONDAY

Totally Tropical Smoothie (see page 41) 213 kcal/16g protein

Watercress, Leek and Pea Soup (see page 44) 200 kcal/ 7.6g protein

Blueberry and Almond Butter Smoothie (see page 36) 200 kcal/20g protein

Greek Salad with Dill and Mint (see page 62) 128 kcal/3.4g protein

Total: 741 kcal/ 47g protein

TUESDAY

Strawberry Shortcake Shake (see page 38) 253kcal/21g protein

Almond and Celeriac Soup (see page 46) 223kcal/7.2g protein

Frozen Berry, Kefir and Vanilla Smoothie (see page 42) 192kcal/ 19g protein

Tangy Courgette Noodles with Coriander, Chilli, Soy and Sesame (see page 58) 98kcal/3.8g protein

Total: 766 kcal/ 51g protein

WEDNESDAY

Kale Glow Smoothie (see page 43) 241 kcal/30g protein

Almond and Celeriac Soup (see page 46) 223 kcal/7.2g protein

Cream of Asparagus Soup (see page 52) 138 kcal/ 4.5g protein

Crudités (see page 66) with Roasted Beetroot Hummus (see page 71) 73+ 165 kcal/ 3.5+5g protein

Total: 840 kcal/ 50g protein

THURSDAY

Strawberry Shortcake Shake (see page 38) 253kcal/21g protein

Cherry and Chocolate Smoothie (see page 37) 265 kcal/28g

Creamy Mushroom Soup (see page 53) 187 kcal/4.8g protein

Summer Tomato Salad with Salsa Verde (see page 61) 115kcal/ 1.8g protein

Total: 840 kcal/ 55.6g protein

FRIDAY

Blueberry and Almond Butter Smoothie (see page 36) 200 kcal/20g protein

Totally Tropical Smoothie (see page 41) 213 kcal/16g protein

Watercress, Leek and Pea Soup (see page 44) 200 kcal/ 7.6g protein

Crudités (see page 66) with Mackerel and Chive Dip

(see page 69) 73+109kcal/3.5+ 6.9g protein

Total: 795 kcal/ 54g protein

SATURDAY

The Ultimate Green Smoothie (see page 34) 221kcal/ 7.7g protein

Chicken and Miso Noodle Soup (see page 49) 156kcal 24g protein

Frozen Berry, Kefir and Vanilla Smoothie (see page 42) 192kcal/ 19g protein)

Crudités (see page 66) with Kale, Garlic and Avocado Cream (see page 68) 73+ 69 kcal/3.5+1.1g protein

Total: 711 kcal/ 54g protein

SUNDAY

Cherry and Chocolate Smoothie (see page 37) 265 kcal/28g

Kale Glow Smoothie (see page 43) 241 kcal/30g protein

Roasted Tomato and Red Pepper Soup (see page 50) 149 kcal/3g protein

Tangy Courgette Noodles with Coriander, Chilli, Soy and Sesame (see page 58) 98kcal/3.8g protein

Total: 753 kcal/ 54g protein

STEP 2

In this Step you are going to start by replacing one shake with a solid meal. The easiest way to do this is to add some protein (such as some meat, fish or a vegetarian alternative) to one of your favourite salads. Once you are comfortable with the reintroduction of solid food, you can replace another shake. Once you have replaced all 3 shakes with solid food you will move into Step 3. Remember, you can always go back to Step 1 or repeat Step 2 at any point on your journey.

MONDAY

Strawberry Shortcake Shake (see page 38)

Rocket leaves with 100g (3½oz) chicken breast, ½ avocado and Simple Basil Vinaigrette (see page 79)

Kale Glow Smoothie (see page 43)

TUESDAY

Blueberry and Almond Butter Smoothie (see page 36)

One-pan Veggie Bean Brunch with Eggs (see page 106)

Beetroot, Coconut and Garlic Soup (see page 54)

WEDNESDAY

Frozen Berry, Kefir and Vanilla Smoothie (see page 42)

Greek Salad with Dill and Mint (see page 62), with 1 can sardines, 20g (¾oz) feta cheese and 10g (¼oz) mixed seeds

Blueberry and Almond Butter Smoothie (see page 36)

THURSDAY

Totally Tropical Smoothie (see page 41)

Baked Lemon & Garlic Salmon Parcel (see page 138)

Cherry and Chocolate Smoothie (see page 37)

FRIDAY

Frozen Berry, Kefir and Vanilla Smoothie (see page 42)

Thai Turkey Burgers, Crunchy Slaw (see pages 150)

Strawberry Shortcake Shake (see page 38)

SATURDAY

Blueberry and Almond Butter Smoothie (see page 36)

1 portion of Roasted Vegetable Quiche with a Cheddar Crust (see page 130) with a handful of salad leaves and a drizzle of balsamic vinegar

Almond and Celeriac Soup (see page 46)

SUNDAY

Totally Tropical Smoothie (see page 41)

Chickpea Dal with Flatbread (see page 129)

Roasted Tomato and Red Pepper Soup (see page 50)

STEP 3

At this stage you should feel in full control, enjoying food and be able to eat socially again. Be mindful of correct portion sizes, and continue to build the healthy habits you have learned. Having lost weight, you are likely to require about a quarter less food than you were previously eating. Many of the Step 3 recipes in this book serve four, so you can enjoy them with friends and family or portion them up and put in the refrigerator for another day.

MONDAY

2 slices of Five-Ingredient Fibre Bread (see page 174) with 2 boiled eggs and sliced avocado

Peanut-Roasted Chicken in Romaine Boats (see p.154)

Fish Pie with Celeriac and Broccoli Topping (see p. 144)

TUESDAY

Overnight berry pot (see page 110)

An open sandwich (2 slices of bread) with Roasted Beetroot Hummus (see page 71), rocket leaves and (¾oz) feta cheese

Perfect Steak with Mushroom Pepper Sauce (see p. 146)

WEDNESDAY

Perfect Soft-Boiled 'Jammy' Eggs with Chilli and Almond Butter (see page 96)

Tangy Courgette Noodles with Coriander, Chilli, Soy and Sesame (see page 58)

Roasted Butternut with Broccoli Pesto (see page 116 – save the other half for lunch tomorrow)

Creamy No-Bake Lemon Cheesecake Pot (see p. 189)

THURSDAY

2 slices of Five-Ingredient Fibre Bread, toasted (see page 174) with butter and No-Sugar Blackberry Jam (see page 184)
Roasted Butternut (leftover from Wednesday), with a rocket salad, 1 can of tuna and Simple Basil Vinaigrette (see page 79)

Lamb Koftas (see page 152) with Greek Salad with Dill and Mint (see page 62) and (¾oz) feta cheese

Fruit and Nut Parfait (see page 183)

FRIDAY

Apple and Cinnamon Omelette (see page 92)

Creamy Courgette Carbonara (see page 149)

Egg-Fried Chicken Cauliflower 'Rice' (see page 159)

Two-Ingredient Chocolate Mousse (see page 186)

SATURDAY

Sweet Strawberry and Almond Frittata (see page 101)

Spinach and Ricotta Stuffed Mushrooms (see page 117)

Marinated Chicken Kebabs (see page 157) with Smoky Sweet Potato Fries (see page 124) and salad leaves

SUNDAY

Spinach, Leek and Feta Omelette (see page 95)

Beetroot, Coconut and Garlic Soup (see page 54) with a slice of Five-Ingredient Fibre Bread (see page 174)

Roast Chicken (see page 166) with a Low-Carb Yorkshire Pudding (see page 168), Roasted Celeriac and Rosemary Roasties (see page 169) and some Creamed Spinach (see page 170).

Blackberry and Almond Crumble (see page 201)

Your meal plan

Over to you!

This page is dedicated to you, so use it to make your own meal plan with your favourite recipes and most successful combinations.

MONDAY

Recipe:

Recipe:

Recipe:

TUESDAY

Recipe:

Recipe:

Recipe:

WEDNESDAY

Recipe:

Recipe:

Recipe:

THURSDAY

Recipe:

Recipe:

Recipe:

FRIDAY

Recipe:

Recipe:

Recipe:

SATURDAY

Recipe:

Recipe:

Recipe:

SUNDAY

Recipe:

Recipe:

Recipe:

INDEX

US / UK GLOSSARY

beetroot	beet	grill	broiler
cannellini beans	white kidney beans	oats	rolled oats
celeriac	celery root	pak choi	bok choi
chickpeas	garbanzo	pepper (red, green)	bell pepper
cordial	fruit syrup	pine nuts	pinyon nuts
coriander	cilantro	sirloin steak	rump steak
courgette	zucchini	spring onion	scallion
desiccated coconut	shredded coconut	soured cream	sour cream
double cream	heavy cream	swede	rutabaga
gherkins	pickles	tin (cake)	cake pan

AUTHOR'S ACKNOWLEDGEMENTS

To my incredible daughters, Florence and Clemmie, the thieves of my heart, my biggest supporters and the most honest taste testers. Being your mother is such a privilege and you are my absolute reason for striving to have the best blood sugar control I can. To my dedicated husband (another loyal taste tester!) and parenting co-pilot, I couldn't have written this book without you. Huge thanks also to my wonderful devoted and supportive parents.

A special thanks to Professor Roy Taylor for believing in my recipes and the vision of this book. For providing the foreword and for giving me so much of your time – it has been a huge privilege and highlight working with you.

To the most exceptional team who brought this book to life: Helena Sutcliffe and Joanna Copestick, Jo Morrell, Sybella Stephens, Lucy Bannell, Nicky Collings, Clare Winfield, Julie Patmore, Kathy Kordalis, Gigi Arnold and Allison Gonsalves – thank you.

There will never be enough words, but, to Jaime, for believing in me. All authors say their agent is the best, but mine really is – I can't thank you enough.

An enormous thanks to my dear friends for their support and encouragement, most notably to Dr Ian Lake, Philip Yates, Polly Mann, Jane Hall McLean, Harriet Mcquoid, Rachel Johnson and Bunty Howe. And to Shannon Andrews for encouraging me to understand the importance of calories!

And that leaves me with you, my wonderful readers, old and new. To those who have attended my talks, my cooking classes and followed me on social media – thank you. If I had known 20 years ago when I was diagnosed with type 1 diabetes that all these years later I would be writing a book to help others living with it, I wouldn't have believed it! Diabetes is a hard disease, it is 24–7 / 365 days a year. It can feel relentless and isolating, but I hope this book and the recipes in it will inspire whole families, help those living with diabetes, give hope and be a permanent fixture in your kitchen.